The Patient-Centered Approach to Medical Note-Writing

AF167523

Christopher J. Wong • Sara L. Jackson
Editors

The Patient-Centered Approach to Medical Note-Writing

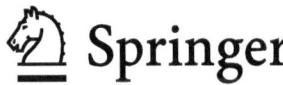 Springer

Editors
Christopher J. Wong
Division of General Internal Medicine
Department of Medicine
University of Washington
Seattle, WA, USA

Sara L. Jackson
Division of General Internal Medicine
Department of Medicine
University of Washington
Seattle, WA, USA

ISBN 978-3-031-43632-1   ISBN 978-3-031-43633-8   (eBook)
https://doi.org/10.1007/978-3-031-43633-8

© The Editor(s) (if applicable) and The Author(s), under exclusive license to Springer Nature Switzerland AG 2023
This work is subject to copyright. All rights are solely and exclusively licensed by the Publisher, whether the whole or part of the material is concerned, specifically the rights of translation, reprinting, reuse of illustrations, recitation, broadcasting, reproduction on microfilms or in any other physical way, and transmission or information storage and retrieval, electronic adaptation, computer software, or by similar or dissimilar methodology now known or hereafter developed.
The use of general descriptive names, registered names, trademarks, service marks, etc. in this publication does not imply, even in the absence of a specific statement, that such names are exempt from the relevant protective laws and regulations and therefore free for general use.
The publisher, the authors, and the editors are safe to assume that the advice and information in this book are believed to be true and accurate at the date of publication. Neither the publisher nor the authors or the editors give a warranty, expressed or implied, with respect to the material contained herein or for any errors or omissions that may have been made. The publisher remains neutral with regard to jurisdictional claims in published maps and institutional affiliations.

This Springer imprint is published by the registered company Springer Nature Switzerland AG
The registered company address is: Gewerbestrasse 11, 6330 Cham, Switzerland

Paper in this product is recyclable.

The editors dedicate this book to:

the visionary founders of the Open Notes movement

our patients who partner with us in their care

our medical students, residents, and fellows, who push themselves and us to always do better for our patients

our colleagues who make work a joy

and all those who helped get us through the pandemic years

Acknowledgments

We would like to thank Sabrina Lai for administrative assistance in creating this book.

Contents

Contributors

Sheida Aalami, MD Division of General Internal Medicine, Department of Medicine, University of Washington, Seattle, WA, USA

Jessica Bender, MD, MPH Division of General Internal Medicine, Department of Medicine, University of Washington, Seattle, WA, USA

Russell Berg, MD, PhD Division of General Internal Medicine, Department of Medicine, University of Washington, Seattle, WA, USA

Rebecca D. Ellis, MD Division of General Internal Medicine, Department of Medicine, University of Washington, Seattle, WA, USA

Cody Gehring, MD Division of General Internal Medicine, Department of Medicine, University of Washington, Seattle, WA, USA

Jeremiah Grams, BS Seattle University, Seattle, WA, USA

Anna F. Hagan, MD Division of General Internal Medicine, Department of Medicine, University of Washington, Seattle, WA, USA

Scott Hagan, MD Division of General Internal Medicine, Department of Medicine, University of Washington, Seattle, WA, USA

Margaret Isaac, MD Division of General Internal Medicine, Department of Medicine, University of Washington, Seattle, WA, USA

Sara L. Jackson, MD, MPH, FACP Division of General Internal Medicine, Department of Medicine, University of Washington, Seattle, WA, USA

Jocelyn James, MD Division of General Internal Medicine, Department of Medicine, University of Washington, Seattle, WA, USA

Jared W. Klein, MD, MPH Division of General Internal Medicine, Department of Medicine, University of Washington, Seattle, WA, USA

Sarah Leyde, MD Division of General Internal Medicine, Department of Medicine, University of Washington, Seattle, WA, USA

Kim O'Connor, MD, MACP Division of General Internal Medicine, Department of Medicine, University of Washington, Seattle, WA, USA

Angad P. Singh, MD Department of Family Medicine, University of Washington, Seattle, WA, USA

Department of Biomedical Informatics and Medical Education, University of Washington, Seattle, WA, USA

Sarah Steinkruger, MD Division of General Internal Medicine, Department of Medicine, University of Washington, Seattle, WA, USA

Renata Thronson, MD, FACP Division of General Internal Medicine, Department of Medicine, University of Washington, Seattle, WA, USA

Christopher J. Wong, MD, FACP Division of General Internal Medicine, Department of Medicine, University of Washington, Seattle, WA, USA

Jennifer Wright, MD, FACP Division of General Internal Medicine, Department of Medicine, University of Washington, Seattle, WA, USA

Part I
Introduction, History, General Principles

Chapter 1
Introduction

Christopher J. Wong and Sara L. Jackson

1.1 Why This Book?

Somewhere the practice of medicine lost its way.

Our collective mission as healthcare professionals is to help our patients—to prevent illnesses from occurring, to treat what is treatable when medical conditions do arise, to support patients through afflictions that are incurable, and to always maintain our patients' dignity and humanity.

And yet, despite what should be the compassionate mindset of those who choose a career in healthcare, harmful language practices have permeated medicine. How did the art of healing transform into terms such as *frequent flyer* and *IV drug abuser*?

We can postulate many possibilities: stress of the job; a punishing training system; excessive workload; the use of humor—however dark—as a means to cope with the moral injury of working in modern-day medicine;[1] or the reinforcement of being in a privileged group that has its own secret lingo. The causes of using harmful language by those who should be healers may differ between healthcare professionals; and of course not everyone has fallen under this stigmatizing spell.

When it comes to writing notes, language that is harmful to patients is frequently used. Much of this language has become so pervasive that providers may not even

---

[1] We are writing this from the United States, which lacks a universal health system.

C. J. Wong (✉) · S. L. Jackson
Division of General Internal Medicine, Department of Medicine, University of Washington, Seattle, WA, USA
e-mail: cjwong@uw.edu; sljack@uw.edu

© The Author(s), under exclusive license to Springer Nature Switzerland AG 2023
C. J. Wong, S. L. Jackson (eds.), *The Patient-Centered Approach to Medical Note-Writing*, https://doi.org/10.1007/978-3-031-43633-8_1

recognize it as stigmatizing or harmful. Our goal in writing this book is to have a resource for anyone who writes medical notes to consider what they are writing with the patient in mind. For many, this will mean unlearning what has been taught either explicitly or implicitly by the medical profession. We expect that some readers will find our recommendations surprising, while others will see them as long overdue.

Beyond improving written language practices, a secondary goal is to improve the professionalism of how we speak as a medical culture. We focus on written notes because not only do patients read them now, but they are also part of the enduring medical record. Some terms are more frequently spoken than written and are so pejorative that we will not even write them here in order not to perpetuate them further [1, 2]. But we do hope that there will be a synergy between our written and oral discourse—that by improving our notes, we will elevate our speech as well.

Finally, we believe there is a training gap; although patients have been able to access notes for a number of years, we continue to see notes that contain language that is not patient-centered. Medical trainees report low levels of education about writing patient-facing notes [3]. We hope that this book can be used to assist others who teach current and future healthcare professionals.

In this era of high-tech medicine, words still matter—it is not only disease and illness that can wound, or medicines and surgeries that can heal.

1.2   The Open Notes Movement

The documentation of medical care has changed dramatically in the last 20 years (see also Chap. 2). Those of us who have been in practice longer recall the era of paper medical charts. Outpatient offices usually had a room that resembled a library, with charts stacked in shelves and pulled when a patient came in for an appointment. Inpatient charts were stored and had to be requested to be reviewed. Patients had significant barriers to accessing their own records, having to go in person to the medical records department and file a request, often incurring fees.

Even having the chart was no panacea, as handwriting often limited the ability to quickly find information, and there was no easy way to trend laboratory tests. Charts lacked a search function as we are accustomed to using with modern electronic health records (EHRs) and search engines.

The electronic health record and the "Open Notes" movement changed everything.

A pioneering study of Open Notes was published in the Annals of Internal Medicine in 2012 [4]. Dr. Tom Delbanco and colleagues invited patients to read their notes at primary care practices in three different healthcare systems in the United States. The vast majority of patients who participated felt that they were better able to understand their health conditions, remember the care plan, be prepared for visits, and feel more in control of their care. Patients had more concerns regarding privacy and confidentiality, while primary care providers had more concerns that Open Notes would cause a patient to feel worried or offended. Notably, over 25% of providers responded that they changed the way they documented as a result.

In a large follow-up survey seven or more years after Open Notes were available, patients reported that access to notes was important for their health management, that they shared the notes frequently with others, and patients from populations that are less well served by the country's healthcare system were more likely to report benefit from access to notes [5]. Benefits of Open Notes also include patients identifying errors when reading their own notes, with the potential to prevent medical errors and improve the quality and safety of healthcare delivery [6].

Concerns about specific populations gaining access to notes, such as those with mental health conditions [7] and adolescent patients [8], have been managed with a combination of open discussion with patients about the contents, thereby building trust and increasing engagement, and at times opting not to share sensitive notes with patients and/or proxies. Additionally, efficient communication with care providers [9], who are critical components of the patient's team, is another reason to actively share notes. Continued assessment of outcomes and best practices in these areas is ongoing.

In the decade following Open Notes, over 50 million patients gained access to their notes as health systems adopted Open Notes based upon the benefits reported in the original trial and patient advocacy. On April 5, 2021, Open Notes became law in the United States after implementation of the Cures Act (Interoperability, Information Blocking, and the Office of the National Coordinator for Health IT Certification Program Final Rule) of the 21st Century Cures Act [10], passed by the US Congress in 2016. The Cures Rule requires all patients to be provided access to all the health information in their electronic health records without charge by their healthcare provider. This includes access to test results that were not part of the original note-sharing studies. Early data suggest that note volume and time spent documenting by clinicians since the Cures Rule went into effect have not changed [11].

Future directions for Open Notes include inviting patients to co-write notes and potentially decrease clinician documentation burden. Telehealth visits may be particularly suited to this co-writing scenario. Early pilot projects with co-generated notes [12], and with OurDX [13], a collaborative online diagnosis tool, suggest increased patient engagement.

Inviting patients into the electronic health record engages them in their health and has the potential to improve healthcare quality and safety. The words that physicians choose are now visible to patients and can in the best circumstances strengthen the therapeutic relationship or, in the worst outcome, strain or even fracture it [14]. This transparency forces healthcare professionals to reflect carefully on how they have documented patient care in the past and to take greater care in documentation moving forward with the knowledge that patients will be reading their own medical chart, often in quasi-real time.

1.3   Patients Are Reading—and Concerned By What They Read

Some providers may read this book and wonder if it is relevant, as they may have note-sharing with patients but so far experienced few, if any, patient complaints.

However, as with many aspects of life, silence does not equal consent or agreement. It is highly likely that patients take issue with aspects of their medical notes far more than they actually mention it to a provider or administrator. In one study of 22,959 patients, 10.5% reported feeling judged or offended by something in the notes [14]—however, healthcare providers probably do not have the real-world experience of one in ten patients asking to address an issue with their notes (if so, providers would likely change their habits quickly!). Another study found that 45.6% of patients found at least one error in their problem list, but of those patients, only 3.5% had asked their provider to correct it [15].

Patient concerns with their medical notes are therefore likely to be underreported. Although these studies did not evaluate reasons for not bringing up note-related concerns, there may be many reasons for this discrepancy, including the power dynamic between provider and patient that may disincentivize patients to speak up. Providers should recognize that just because a patient is not actively objecting to something written in their chart, it does not mean that they agree with it, or that they have not been harmed, or that the patient-provider relationship has not been affected, or that the trust in the overall healthcare system has not been diminished. Therefore, it is the responsibility of healthcare professionals who write notes to not wait for patients to raise issues, but rather to be trained in and practice patient-centered documentation.

1.4   Conventions Used in This Book

As a book about language, we should start with some basic conventions about language that we have chosen to use.

1.4.1   Pronouns

When using examples in which gender does not matter to the example, we have made the decision to use *they* as a singular third-person pronoun and correspondingly *their* and *them* when appropriate. For example: *The patient returns today to discuss their hypertension. They are taking all their medications and report home blood readings of 120/80 on average.* We felt that using a default gender of either *he* or *she* would create gender bias. Some authors use *he or she*, but we felt that doing so would not only create more awkward writing than simply using *they* but would also exclude patients who use other pronouns.

We recognize that many of our patients do not identify with either a male or female gender, or they use other pronoun words. While to some readers we acknowledge that it may seem jarring to see the singular use of "they," we believe that this is a useful convention, as well as a potential evolutionary trend in the English language in general (in some languages there simply is no gendered pronoun at all).

Therefore, in most examples in this book, the use of *they* will represent a neutral third-person pronoun, and not imply that the example is of a patient who uses *they* as a nonbinary pronoun. When gender is an important part of the discussion, then that will be specifically addressed in the chapter, and other pronouns may be used in the examples (see Chap. 4 for the discussion of gender and Chap. 7 for the discussion of its inclusion in the one-liner or identifying statement in a note).

1.4.2 Fonts and Quotations

One educational challenge when writing a book about writing is that we will need to show examples. There are a few ways to do this: using quotations, changing fonts such as using *italics*, or offsetting the example text in either a table or separate paragraph. Because the use of quotations is one of the examples of potentially doubting language (used in multiple parts of a chart; see Chaps. 3 and 7), when using text examples within a paragraph, we decided in general not to show text in quotes, but to use italics instead, as italics are less frequently used in medical chart notes (although in an EHR note writers have control over fonts such as color, bold typeface, and italics, it is often an extra step to do so and in our experience less commonly used). When example text is shown in a table or in a separate paragraph, we will show this text without quotations or italics.

1.4.3 Names

Some authors use generic names such as *John Smith* or *Mary Jones*. There is no easy way around the bias toward names that are congruent with certain ethnic or ancestral backgrounds. We considered using a wide variety of common names from different cultures but ultimately determined that there is no good way of doing so. Instead, we will use a blank line _____ or, when pertinent, brackets where a name would be located in a chart note: e.g., *Dear* _____ or *Dear* [*First Name*] [*Last Name*].

1.4.4 Brackets

When showing language in which there are words or phrases that do not need a specific text example, or for which an example would not be appropriate, we will use brackets. As noted in the example above using a patient's name, rather than making up a name, we will use brackets to denote content of text rather than the actual words themselves.

1.4.5 We and You

We will mostly use third person, but as in this chapter, we at times may directly address the reader. In those instances, *we* refers to the chapter authors and the editors, and *you* refers to the intended audience of healthcare professionals.

1.4.6 Terms

EHR We will use EHR to refer to the electronic health record rather than EMR.

Person-First Language This term refers to the concept of putting a person first, before their medical or social condition. An example is: a *person with diabetes* rather than a *diabetic*. Person-first language has been used to speak more respectfully about people with disabilities [16] and in the field of psychiatry [17]. As will be noted in chapters that follow, patients themselves may have different preferences about how they wish to be addressed—for advocacy, condition-first (or disease-first or disability-first) language can be useful for solidarity and organizing. For an individual patient's chart note, we recommend person-first language as a default but also to engage with patients as individuals as to their preferences.

Healthcare Professional, Clinician, Provider, or Note Writer When referring to people who write medical notes about patients, we will use these terms. We are deliberately using these terms as interchangeable and all-encompassing. We recognize that there are many terms for healthcare professionals (e.g., doctor, physician, surgeon, nurse, medical assistant, nurse practitioner, physical therapist, pharmacist) and that terms vary between countries and regions. For the purposes of education about patient-centered notes, all of these professionals may interact with patients and document in the medical record.

Patient-Centered We find the following description of patient-centered care to be useful: "In patient-centered care, an individual's specific health needs and desired health outcomes are the driving force behind all health care decisions and quality measurements. Patients are partners with their health care providers, and providers treat patients not only from a clinical perspective, but also from an emotional, mental, spiritual, social, and financial perspective" [18]. Patient-centered *documentation* ideally represents patient-centered *care*, and not simply a rewording of poorly delivered healthcare. It is our belief that using patient-centered *language* is synergistic with and promotes patient-centered *care*.

Open Notes   We will use Open Notes as a general term for medical chart notes that are viewable by patients. The organization OpenNotes (https://www.opennotes.org), written as one word, is a group of collaborators who have researched and advocated for transparency in healthcare, including chart notes.

Patient-Facing   This term refers to anyone or anything that has a direct interaction with a patient. For example, a phlebotomist who draws blood from a patient is patient-facing, whereas a laboratory technologist who runs tests on the sample (without seeing the patient) is not. For the EHR, not only chart notes but also other aspects of the chart may be patient-facing, including problem lists (Chap. 8), medicine lists, test results (Chap. 15), direct communications (Chap. 17), and diagnostic codes.

1.5   Language Evolves

Language is a living, changing entity. It varies by a number of factors and can change both slowly and quickly. Definitions of words can change; new words can be created; new meanings for old words can emerge; and other words can fade out of use. Not only words but also grammar and punctuation evolve as well.

The recommendations in this book will vary in strength. Some practices we feel are not right and strongly urge note writers to follow: e.g., do not include race as part of an objective physical examination. Other recommendations are more stylistic and may vary by context: e.g., the use of quotations can be negative (doubting the patient's history or beliefs) or positive (giving voice to a patient). Some recommended language may change over time or lack consensus as to their relative value or stigma: e.g., some people view *nonadherent* as less stigmatizing than *noncompliant*, but others may view both as equally pejorative and unnecessary.

This book is not meant as simply a list of dos and don'ts. Nor is it meant to be an oppressive means to damper anyone's speech. Rather, as the examples will show, more often than not, relatively simple changes in language can be more medically accurate and at the same time more patient-centered.

1.6   Scope of This Book

Because we are discussing matters related specifically to language, we focus on English-language chart documentation. We anticipate that similar concerns may arise in other languages that are beyond the scope of this book. Other locations of healthcare practice may have different issues of bias, as bias is a cultural phenomenon. The English language is varied within and among different countries; therefore, some of the data cited may not be generalizable outside of the region or country in which a study was conducted. While many of the seminal literature studies were conducted in the United States, commentaries suggest that similar language issues exist outside the United States [19–21].

For this edition of the book, we are focusing on medical notes and are not addressing procedural notes specifically. We also focus on adult medical care and for this edition are not reviewing issues specific to the pediatric population. However, the principles of patient-centered note writing are universal.

We have organized this book to contain chapters on general principles but also individual sections of the medical chart so that readers can read a chapter in isolation should they choose.

Part I: Introduction, History, and General Principles

In addition to this introductory chapter, we review the history and goals of medical charts and the general principles pertaining to patient-centered language and discuss the use of electronic health record.

Chapter 2: Goals of Medical Notes and Records

This chapter reviews a brief history of medical documentation from ancient times to the present. It then reviews the goals of medical charts—what they are for and how they have evolved over time. Notably, charts serve multiple roles, making a provider's task challenging.

Chapter 3: General Principles: Language, Bias, and Harmful Notes

In this chapter we address core issues of bias, language, and the ways in which language can potentially be harmful to patients. We discuss some of the seminal work of Park et al. [22] in categorizing types of positive and negative language and review the literature regarding inequal distribution of negative or stigmatizing language. We present a framework on how biased language and chart notes create a cycle that can affect patients and become self-perpetuating. The stigmatizing language themes discussed in this chapter will be repeated throughout this book to varying degrees. For example, labeling is a common theme, and will be discussed most in Chap. 7, where the identification statement is often the first source of biasing the reader. Stigmatizing diagnostic codes are addressed in both the Problem List (Chap. 8) and Assessment and Plan (Chap. 13) chapters.

Chapter 4: General Principles: Race, Ethnicity, and Gender

This chapter addresses the often-problematic topics of race, ethnicity, and gender. Race and ethnicity may be important for some parts of the medical note (e.g., the Social History), but not others (e.g., the identification statement or "one-liner"). Furthermore, race and ethnicity are often incorrectly portrayed as biological rather than social constructs. Gender terminology is reviewed. Gender is a complex topic for which clinicians should work with their patients as to their correct gender and gender-related terms.

Chapter 5: General Principles: Body Habitus and What Is "Normal"

Body habitus and the words used to describe it are often laden with bias and can be a source of stigma. A related concept is what *normal* means in medicine—the many ways it is used and potentially misused.

Chapter 6: The Electronic Health Record

The electronic health record is rapidly becoming ubiquitous. The principles of patient-centered language can occur verbally, with hand-written text, and with the EHR. The EHR, however, has the ability to facilitate (or hinder) the use of patient-centered language. This chapter addresses design techniques in which the EHR can promote best practices, using the SOAP (Subjective, Objective, Assessment, and Plan) note framework.

Part II: The Medical Note

In this next section, we address individual parts of a typical medical note and how patient-centered language can be used in each.

Chapter 7: The Chief "Complaint" and History of Present Illness

This chapter reviews the identification statement, the Chief Complaint, and the history of present illness (HPI). The authors cover the fact that a "chief complaint" is not a particularly accurate term, and is no longer required for medical billing using this specific phrase, which was one of the previous drivers for use of the term. They challenge some of the recalcitrant traditions in medicine such as including information in the identification statement that not only may not be necessary but is also often stigmatizing. They discuss the use of doubting language in the HPI and offer more patient-centered alternatives.

Chapter 8: The Problem List and Past Medical History

Here we delve into the Problem List, a term ingrained in the minds of many clinicians but which deserves a closer look. The chapter discusses the origins of the Problem List, and the varied elements it may include, such as past (resolved) problems, risk factors, and other conditions that may not be strictly "problems." Coding terminology is often outdated, and alternatives may be used.

Chapter 9: The Social History

In this chapter, the Social History is reviewed. Varied in purpose, it may include race, ethnicity, gender, marital status and family structure, substance use, sexual health, housing status, incarceration history, occupation, and language preference, among a myriad of other subjects that do not traditionally reside in other parts of the medical note. These topics are frequent sources of potentially harmful language.

Chapter 10: Substance Use and Substance Use Disorders

While many of the same principles apply to substance use and substance use disorders as are discussed in other chapters, for these conditions in particular the use of stigmatizing language is pervasive. In addition to the practice of labeling patients either as their condition or using pejorative language, discussion of substance use also frequently uses terminology associated with failure and policing. This chapter addresses stigmatizing terminology frequently used in the context of substance use and provides recommendations for more patient-centered alternatives.

Chapter 11: Mental Health

For documentation of mental health, there is a distinction between a well-done mental status exam by a psychiatrist and potentially problematic descriptions by nonpsychiatrists, especially in the history of present illness and the physical exam. For patients who are at a high risk of being harmed from reading their notes, the current regulations in the United States do allow for limited situations in which providers can choose to not share a note with a patient.

Chapter 12: The Review of Systems and the Physical Examination

Stigmatizing language is frequently found in the Review of Systems and Physical Examination. This chapter discusses the effect of billing and coding requirements on documentation and how updated guidelines can allow for more patient-centered notes with less "note bloat."

Chapter 13: The Assessment and Plan

The Assessment and Plan occupies a higher place of importance in the medical note, as it is often the first (or only) part of the note that other healthcare professionals read. Importantly, one-liners may return in the Assessment and Plan and may serve as an initial statement biasing the reader. Language can greatly affect how each item in the Assessment and Plan is written, including how conditions are named, how well they are controlled, and whether a patient responds to treatment. The Assessment and Plan is particularly well suited to shared decision-making language and resonates poorly when non-partnering language is used instead.

Chapter 14: Difficult Encounters

The authors of this chapter tackle a topic of great importance: the Difficult Encounter (a better term than *difficult patient*). No matter how well we perform as clinicians, at some point we will have a difficult interaction with a patient. This chapter addresses some of the ways that the stigmatizing language discussed in the previous chapters can be even more important to recognize after a difficult encounter. Common challenging documentation situations are discussed, including being doubted, disagreements with patients, being challenged or accused, and when a patient exhibits inappropriate behavior. The authors propose a framework for difficult encounters in order to create documentation that is accurate but not pejorative.

Part III: Other Note Types and Presentations

While the focus of this book is on the medical note, with the modern-day EHR, there is so much functionality that it is an entire environment in which we write text in multiple formats and for multiple purposes, nearly all of which is able to be seen by our patients. Finally, we would be remiss not to at least acknowledge the interaction between our verbal language and our written language.

Chapter 15: Tests and Studies

This chapter discusses a topic practiced daily yet seldom taught: how to communicate test results to patients in the EHR, paying attention to how to address the patient, what to write, and how to handle potentially serious results in the era of auto-released results.

Chapter 16: Oral Case Presentations

While this topic may seem far afield from note writing, the authors demonstrate the connections between what we say and what we write. The oral case presentation is a verbal form of the written note and is subject to similar language issues. The live aspect of an oral presentation in front of a patient requires additional considerations, including the ability to gauge a patient's reactions and interact in real time. Moreover, some language issues are magnified by speaking them aloud in front of a patient, especially labeling. Additionally, when engaging in verbal discussions of patients, an argument is made for always maintaining patient-centered, non-stigmatizing language, whether a patient is present or not.

Chapter 17: Care Outside of the Clinical Encounter: Electronic Communications and Documentation of Telephone Calls

Care of patients, especially in the ambulatory setting, often occurs outside of a face-to-face clinical encounter. Healthcare professionals now frequently respond to emails or other electronic communications and must learn how to do so in a patient-centered manner. Clinicians must now adjust to the possibility that documentation of telephone calls may be visible to patients, leading to reconsideration of what is entered into them.

1.7 Conclusion

Patients accessing their electronic health record is here to stay, including previously unavailable parts of their charts such as test results and telephone notes. Research is actively being done as to the prevalence and types of potentially stigmatizing language contained in chart notes. Education regarding how best to document in the era of "Open Notes" remains a work in progress. With this book we hope not only to add to the resources available to improve notes for our patients but also to improve the culture of medicine as a whole to make it more patient-centered. We recognize that language will continue to evolve, and, as healthcare professionals, we need to evolve with it to provide the best care for our patients.

References

1. Dans PE. The use of pejorative terms to describe patients: "Dirtball" revisited. Proc (Bayl Univ Med Cent). 2002;15(1):26–30. https://doi.org/10.1080/08998280.2002.11927811.
2. Goldman B. Derogatory slang in the hospital setting. AMA J Ethics. 2015;17(2):167–71. https://doi.org/10.1001/virtualmentor.2015.17.2.msoc2-1502.
3. Schiller PT, Wong CJ, Golob AL, Kimel-Scott K, Sobel HG, Pasanen ME, Pincavage AT. Internal medicine intern preparedness to document clinical encounters in the era of open notes: a needs assessment survey. J Gen Intern Med. 2023;38(6):1556–8. https://doi.org/10.1007/s11606-023-08099-2.
4. Delbanco T, Walker J, Bell SK, Darer JD, Elmore JG, Farag N, Feldman HJ, Mejilla R, Ngo L, Ralston JD, Ross SE, Trivedi N, Vodicka E, Leveille SG. Inviting patients to read their doctors'

notes: a quasi-experimental study and a look ahead. Ann Intern Med. 2012;157(7):461–70. Erratum in: Ann Intern Med. 2015;162(7):532. https://doi.org/10.7326/0003-4819-157-7 -201210020-00002.

5. Walker J, Leveille S, Bell S, Chimowitz H, Dong Z, Elmore JG, Fernandez L, Fossa A, Gerard M, Fitzgerald P, Harcourt K, Jackson S, Payne TH, Perez J, Shucard H, Stametz R, DesRoches C, Delbanco T. OpenNotes after 7 years: patient experiences with ongoing access to their clinicians' outpatient visit notes. J Med Internet Res. 2019;21(5):e13876. Erratum in: J Med Internet Res. 2020;22(4):e18639. https://doi.org/10.2196/13876.

6. Bell SK, Delbanco T, Elmore JG, Fitzgerald PS, Fossa A, Harcourt K, Leveille SG, Payne TH, Stametz RA, Walker J, DesRoches CM. Frequency and types of patient-reported errors in electronic health record ambulatory care notes. JAMA Netw Open. 2020;3(6):e205867. https://doi.org/10.1001/jamanetworkopen.2020.5867.

7. Schwarz J, Bärkås A, Blease C, Collins L, Hägglund M, Markham S, Hochwarter S. Sharing clinical notes and electronic health records with people affected by mental health conditions: scoping review. JMIR Ment Health. 2021;8(12):e34170. https://doi.org/10.2196/34170.

8. Lam B, Bourgeois F, DesRoches C, et al. Attitudes, experiences, and safety behaviours of adolescents and young adults who read visit notes: opportunities to engage patients early in their care. Future Healthc J. 2021;8(3):e585–92. https://doi.org/10.7861/fhj.2021-0118.

9. Jackson SL, Shucard H, Liao JM, Bell SK, Fossa A, Payne TH, Reisch LM, Radick AC, DesRoches CM, Fitzgerald P, Leveille S, Walker J, Elmore JG. Care partners reading patients' visit notes via patient portals: characteristics and perceptions. Patient Educ Couns. 2022;105(2):290–6. https://doi.org/10.1016/j.pec.2021.08.025.

10. HealthIT.gov. ONC's cures act final rule. https://www.healthit.gov/topic/oncs-cures-act-final-rule. Accessed 10 Apr 2023.

11. Holmgren AJ, Apathy NC. Assessing the impact of patient access to clinical notes on clinician EHR documentation. J Am Med Inform Assoc. 2022;29(10):1733–6. https://doi.org/10.1093/jamia/ocac120.

12. Walker J, Leveille S, Kriegel G, et al. Patients contributing to visit notes: mixed methods evaluation of our notes. J Med Internet Res. 2021;23(11):e29951. https://doi.org/10.2196/29951.

13. Bell S, Bourgeois F, Liu S, Thomas EJ, Lowe E, Salmi L. Co-development of OurDX—an online tool to facilitate patient and family engagement in the diagnostic process. BMJ Opin. 2021. https://blogs.bmj.com/bmj/2021/10/14/co-development-of-ourdx-an-online-tool-to-facilitate-patient-and-family-engagement-in-the-diagnostic-process/. Accessed 15 May 2023.

14. Fernández L, Fossa A, Dong Z, Delbanco T, Elmore J, Fitzgerald P, Harcourt K, Perez J, Walker J, DesRoches C. Words matter: what do patients find judgmental or offensive in outpatient notes? J Gen Intern Med. 2021;36(9):2571–8. https://doi.org/10.1007/s11606-020-06432-7.

15. Wright A, Feblowitz J, Maloney FL, Henkin S, Ramelson H, Feltman J, Bates DW. Increasing patient engagement: patients' responses to viewing problem lists online. Appl Clin Inform. 2014;5(4):930–42. https://doi.org/10.4338/ACI-2014-07-RA-0057.

16. Washington DC Office of Disability Rights. People first language. https://odr.dc.gov/page/people-first-language. Accessed 2 Apr 2023.

17. Eriksson AI, Onalaja D. Use of disempowering language: see people as people first. BMJ. 2022;377:o1418. https://doi.org/10.1136/bmj.o1418.

18. NEJM Catalyst. What is patient-centered care? https://catalyst.nejm.org/doi/full/10.1056/CAT.17.0559. Accessed 3 Apr 2023.

19. Cox C, Fritz Z. Presenting complaint: use of language that disempowers patients. BMJ. 2022;377:e066720. https://doi.org/10.1136/bmj-2021-066720.

20. Bircher R. The language we use causes doctors stress too. BMJ. 2022;377:o1266. https://doi.org/10.1136/bmj.o1266.

21. Lajeunesse M. Language that disempowers patients: the doctor is the poor historian. BMJ. 2022;377:o1296. https://doi.org/10.1136/bmj.o1296.

22. Park J, Saha S, Chee B, Taylor J, Beach MC. Physician use of stigmatizing language in patient medical records. JAMA Netw Open. 2021;4(7):e2117052. https://doi.org/10.1001/jamanetworkopen.2021.17052.

Chapter 2
Goals of Medical Notes and Records

Sara L. Jackson and Christopher J. Wong

2.1 Introduction

Humans have documented medical conditions since the earliest recorded written communication. The goals for this documentation have evolved along with medical knowledge, the systems for recording and organizing the information, and the complexity of the healthcare system (Table 2.1).

S. L. Jackson (✉) · C. J. Wong
Division of General Internal Medicine, Department of Medicine, University of Washington, Seattle, WA, USA
e-mail: sljack@uw.edu; cjwong@uw.edu

© The Author(s), under exclusive license to Springer Nature Switzerland AG 2023
C. J. Wong, S. L. Jackson (eds.), *The Patient-Centered Approach to Medical Note-Writing*, https://doi.org/10.1007/978-3-031-43633-8_2

Table 2.1 Historical epochs and goals of medical writing

Representative landmarks by period	Dates	Goals
Prehistoric period		
Lascaux cave pictograms	17,000–15,000 years ago	Description of illness
Vinča culture—logographic scripts	5500–4000 BCE	
Egyptian, Elamite, Sumerian cultures—cuneiform and hieroglyphic writings	4000–3000 BCE	
Unsystematic documentation		
Papyrus scripts	1700–1600 BCE	Description of diagnosis, evaluation, treatment; education
Corpus Hippocraticum	500–400 BCE	
Schola Medica Salernitana—first medical data archiving in Europe	900–1300	
Systematic paper documentation		
Benjamin Rush, physician—book-like medical records	1745–1813	Description of diagnosis, evaluation, treatment; record for the physician and colleagues; education; scientific inquiry (including data collection); billing; medicolegal; record for payers
Universities in Berlin (Charite) and Paris—systematic medical records	1800	
New York Hospital books of admissions and discharges	1793	
Medical records for insurance in Europe and the United States	1880	
Mayo Clinic—collected data into single patient chart	1907	
American College of Surgeons develops standardized treatment diaries	1919	
Introduction of rules for paper-based records	1940	
Systematic electronic documentation		
Introduction of punch cards for filling in medical data	1960	As per systematic paper documentation, with the addition of communication with patients and caregivers over time
Home-grown electronic health records—early patient portals	1970s–1990s	
HITECH legislation increases US use of EHRs and interactive patient portals	2009	

Adapted from Lorkowski J, Pokorski M. Medical records: a historical narrative. Biomedicines. 2022;10:2594. https://doi.org/10.3390/biomedicines10102594 [Open Access]

2.2   The Early History of Medical Documentation

In the prehistoric period, early human depictions included medical injury, such as a cave painting in the Lascaux cave complex in southwestern France of a person attacked by an animal. The early civilizations such as the Vinča, Egyptian, Elamite, and Sumerian recorded descriptions of health events [1].

Documenting clinical symptoms, physical exam, diagnosis, and treatment for educational purposes followed in Egyptian papyrus treatises from 1600 to 1500 and by Hippocrates of Kos (460–370 BC) and Galen in the Roman era was all foundational. During the Middle Ages, Islamic scholars Rhazes, Avicenna, and the Rabbi Maimonides all produced important texts that informed other healers for educational purposes [1].

When anatomical dissection became more common during the Renaissance, associating clinical characteristics with physiology propelled the scientific understanding of diseases. Leonardo da Vinci's (1452–1529) anatomical drawings and Andreas Vesalius' book *De Humani Corporis Fabrica* (1534) resulted in significant advances in medical understanding. Medical documentation continued to focus on educational purposes, with scientific inquiry burgeoning [1].

2.3   Systematic Paper Documentation

Unsystematic educational reports transitioned to systematic paper records in the eighteenth and nineteenth centuries as academic settings strove to standardize record formats. Physician Benjamin Rush recorded detailed patient data in a book, the format of which is considered the original model for the medical history [2]. Universities in Berlin and Paris used written records of conditions and treatment and details of interesting cases as part of the educational process [1], and in the late 1700s, the New York Hospital began cataloguing admission and discharge data [3]. While written patient data were becoming routine in academic settings, much medical care remained undocumented.

In the twentieth century, more attention began to be paid to the processes of medical documentation. Medical records were considered crucial to quality medical care and education in a report by the Rockefeller Foundation and highlighted in the Abraham Flexner Report of 1910 [4]. The challenge of data dispersion began to be addressed at St. Mary's Clinic and the Mayo Clinic in 1907 by collecting information in a single patient chart [2]. In 1919 the American College of Surgeons standardized criteria for treatment diaries [5], and further systematization of records occurred during the Second World War [2]. The goals for these now more systematized charts included collecting data for scientific inquiry, for payment and insurance, and for medicolegal documentation. The records were, however, often illegible.

2.4 Systematic Electronic Documentation

In the 1960s health data were first entered into computers using punch cards. Electronic records gradually increased in use with advances in computing technology, often in the form of home-grown systems at various medical centers. The early systems had limited capabilities—for example, access to laboratory studies or note-writing, but lacking order entry and patient communication. Widespread adoption of large-scale electronic health record systems with advanced functionality occurred after the passage of the Health Information Technology for Economic and Clinical Health (HITECH) Act in 2009 [6]. The purpose of the legislation was to promote the adoption and "meaningful use" of information technology. Prior to 2009 only 10% of US medical institutions had computerized records, and by 2011 nearly 50% of US physicians used electronic record systems [7]. Patient access to electronic health records has also increased globally, and with variable uptake and processes [8].

2.5 Medical Records Belong to Patients: HIPAA, Open Notes, and the 21st Century Cures Act

Patient access to the medical records was facilitated by the advent of electronic health records, which were legible and more easily shared via electronic portals. In the United States, patients had legal access to their medical records beginning in 1996 when the Health Insurance Portability and Accountability Act (HIPAA) was passed, but copying paper records was time-consuming and required requesting and payment for records.

As electronic systems were rapidly adopted, the Open Notes movement championed patient access to their own medical information [9]. In 2012 a report of the experiences of 105 physicians and 20,000 patients who shared their notes in three health systems found that doctors' workloads did not change; patients resoundingly approved of the practice of note sharing and felt more in control of their health and healthcare; and few patients were worried or confused by reading their notes [10].

In 2021 the 21st Century Cures Act implementation began requiring all US health systems to electronically share clinician notes with patients at no charge for online access [11]. As patients and caregivers are more easily able to access and read their medical notes, the onus is on health systems and physicians to optimize the language and clarity of notes to best communicate key information so that patients are engaged in participating in their healthcare.

2.6 Goals of Medical Charts

Certain goals of medical charts have persisted unchanged since the earliest days, including being a means to describe a patient's illness and preserve it for a future date for others to see and for the education of other healthcare professionals.

However, ancient practitioners of medicine never envisioned billing and coding requirements or emails with patients. The environment of medical charts in the present day has asked the medical note—and therefore the provider—to accomplish many goals, not always consistent with one another.

Billing and coding have undoubtedly influenced the way that notes are written in the United States. Medical notes have for over 20 years been influenced by coding requirements necessary to achieve certain levels of service. These complex incentives affected many parts of the medical note, such as enshrining the "chief complaint" (Chap. 7), and leading many providers to include extensive Review of Systems and Physical Exam elements (Chap. 12), one of the many factors in what is called "note bloat." Unfortunately, adding more sections may lead to questionable documentation, including unnecessary general descriptors and cursorily performed (and documented) parts of the physical examination. New billing rules should reduce this problem but may take time for an ingrained medical culture to adopt.

Providers have had to change the way they document conditions because of coding and its effect on reimbursement. For example, the current generation of providers in the United States has learned to use the awkward phrase *acute blood loss anemia, due to gastrointestinal bleeding*, whereas prior generations would simply have written *GI bleed*. While some terms evolve due to true clinical refinement, others may be forced into medical documentation due to coding requirements such as these.

Other governmental regulatory requirements include having to monitor quality measures. For patients on certain Medicare plans, the Centers for Medicare and Medicaid Services (CMS) requires plans to submit Healthcare Effectiveness Data and Information Set (HEDIS) data reports to the National Committee for Quality Assurance (NCQA) [12]. While not all of these data have to be in a provider note, they are still in the EHR, most of which is now accessible to patients. For example, a patient may have well-treated depression but discover that they have a "care gap" in the EHR because they did not have a follow-up PHQ-9 (Patient Health Questionnaire-9) score documented in the chart [13]. Other requirements such as the Hierarchical Condition Category (HCC) system may steer providers toward potentially harmful language such as when coding for obesity (see Chap. 5).

Thus, providers in the current era find themselves in a potentially stressful situation, as demonstrated in Table 2.2, which lists the many expectations of their

Table 2.2 Multiple motivations and influences affecting medical charts	
	• Description of illness
	• Description of diagnosis, evaluation, treatment
	• Education
	• Scientific inquiry (including data collection)
	• Payment (insurance)
	• Medicolegal
	• Record for the physician and colleagues
	• Transparency to the patient
	• Direct communication with the patient
	• Quality improvement
	• Governmental regulations

documentation. Even if they believe in the principles of transparency for patients, they may be concerned at having to relearn how to write notes knowing that patients will be reading them. While they may look positively toward this challenge, they also face pressures from the regulatory and billing environment to include other language and terms in the chart note, not all of which are patient-centered. And finally, they must still attempt to write a note that is useful to patient care, and also defensible should there be future medicolegal issues, while balancing other competing demands for time.

2.7   Future Charts

There is hope for change. As noted above and in Chaps. 7 and 12, requirements for medical notes have become less burdensome. The Open Notes movement may improve the use of patient-centered language not only in notes patients read but may spread into more respectful discourse in general. Advocacy groups will pressure governmental organizations to change harmful terms.

The next evolution of patient-centered medical charts may be shared notes or entirely patient-created notes. Already patients can now enter a narrative in many EHR systems about what their visit is concerning, effectively constituting their version of the reason for visit and HPI.

Improved EHR design and note templates could potentially return healthcare professionals to writing about what is most important (patient care) in a patient-centered manner.

References

1. Lorkowski J, Pokorski M. Medical records: a historical narrative. Biomedicine. 2022;10:2594. https://doi.org/10.3390/biomedicines10102594.
2. Gillum RF. From papyrus to the electronic tablet: a brief history of the clinical medical record with lessons for the digital age. Am J Med. 2013;126:853–7.
3. Engle RL Jr. The evolution, uses, and present problems of the patient's medical record as exemplified by the records of the New York Hospital from 1793 to the present. Trans Am Clin Climatol Assoc. 1991;102:182–9.
4. Flexner A. Medical Education in the United States and Canada: a report to the Carnegie Foundation for the Advancement of Teaching; Bulletin 4. New York: The Carnegie Foundation for the Advancement of Teaching; 1910. http://archive.carnegiefoundation.org/publications/pdfs/elibrary/Carnegie_Flexner_Report.pdf. Accessed 5 Oct 2023.
5. Timmermans S, Berg M. The gold standard. The challenge of evidence-based medicine and standardization in health care. Philadelphia: Temple University Press; 2003.
6. What is the HITECH Act? The HIPAA Journal. https://www.hipaajournal.com/what-is-the-hitech-act/. Accessed 5 Oct 2023.
7. Berner ES, Detmer DE, Simborg D. Will the wave finally break? A brief view of the adoption of electronic medical records in the United States. J Am Med Inform Assoc. 2005;12(1):3–7. https://doi.org/10.1197/jamia.M1664.

8. Essén A, Scandurra I, Gerrits R, Humphrey G, Johansen MA, Kierkegaard P, Koskinen J, Liaw S, Odeh S, Ross P, Ancker JS. Patient access to electronic health records: differences across ten countries. Health Policy Technol. 2018;7(1):44–56. https://doi.org/10.1016/j.hlpt.2017.11.003.
9. Opennotes. Our history: fifty years in the making. https://www.opennotes.org/history/. Accessed 14 Mar 2023.
10. Delbanco T, Walker J, Bell SK, Darer JD, Elmore JG, Farag N, Feldman HJ, Mejilla R, Ngo L, Ralston JD, Ross SE, Trivedi N, Vodicka E, Leveille SG. Inviting patients to read their doctors' notes: a quasi-experimental study and a look ahead. Ann Intern Med. 2012;157(7):461–70. Erratum in: Ann Intern Med. 2015;162(7):532. https://doi.org/10.7326/0003-4819-157-7-201210020-00002.
11. HealthIT. Information blocking. https://www.healthit.gov/topic/information-blocking. Accessed 14 Mar 2023.
12. Reporting Requirements for HEDIS® Measurement Year (MY) 2022, HOS, and CAHPS® measures, and information regarding HOS and HOS-M for frailty. https://www.cms.gov/files/document/2023reportingrequirementsforhedishosandcahps5182022g.pdf. Accessed 14 Mar 2023.
13. National Committee for Quality Assurance. Utilization of the PHQ-9 to monitor depression symptoms for adolescents and adults (DMS). https://www.ncqa.org/hedis/measures/utilization-of-the-phq-9-to-monitor-depression-symptoms-for-adolescents-and-adults/. Accessed 14 Mar 2023.

Chapter 3
General Principles: Language, Bias, and Harmful Notes

Christopher J. Wong and Sara L. Jackson

3.1 Introduction

When tackling the problem of how to make clinical notes more patient-centered, we must first examine what makes notes *not* patient-centered. This chapter addresses the presence of bias on the part of healthcare professionals, how biased language appears in clinical notes, the disparities in which patients receive more biased language in their notes, and discusses a framework to consider the relationship between note-writing, the patient, and the clinician.

3.2 Bias: Definition and Types

There are many definitions of *bias*. In this book, we refer to bias using the following definition:

Bias
Prejudice in favor of or against one thing, person, or group compared with another, usually in a way considered to be unfair [1].

C. J. Wong (✉) · S. L. Jackson
Division of General Internal Medicine, Department of Medicine, University of Washington, Seattle, WA, USA
e-mail: cjwong@uw.edu; sljack@uw.edu

© The Author(s), under exclusive license to Springer Nature Switzerland AG 2023
C. J. Wong, S. L. Jackson (eds.), *The Patient-Centered Approach to Medical Note-Writing*, https://doi.org/10.1007/978-3-031-43633-8_3

We are not born with biases. Rather, they arise from a complex array of social and environmental factors. In the healthcare setting, biases that are particularly problematic for patients may include assumptions about race, ethnicity, gender, age, social factors, disability, and diseases [2] (Table 3.1).

Biases are often discussed in a negative context—that is, negative treatment of a patient occurs due to a negative bias. This situation is clearly inappropriate, and a goal is to avoid such outcomes. However, positive treatment, when due to bias, is also an undesired and inequitable outcome in healthcare. For example, a healthcare professional may "go the extra mile" for a patient who is perceived positively by the healthcare professional in some manner (Table 3.2).

Table 3.1 Common domains in which bias may arise in healthcare settings[a]

Domain	Example
Age	Assuming an older person is less capable
Gender	Assuming a transgender person has gender dysphoria
Race	Offering fewer pain medications to a patient perceived to be a certain race (*racism*)
Ethnicity	Assuming an occupation about a person based on the person's ethnicity
Behavior	Calling a patient agitated when they are upset or effusive
Health condition	Assuming a patient with a history of substance use disorder is inappropriately asking for pain medications
Disability	Focusing on a patient's disability and assuming that they wish they were not disabled
Class	Assuming a patient has low health literacy by judging their appearance or speech

[a]This list is not meant to be complete—there are additional areas where people can hold biases toward another person

Table 3.2 Examples of positive and negative bias—both types may lead to inequitable care

Type of bias	Biased perception	Biased action
Negative bias	A healthcare professional perceives a patient as inappropriately drug-seeking because of the patient's race	A healthcare professional does not adequately treat a patient's pain
Positive bias	A healthcare professional perceives a patient more favorably because of the patient's class and status (e.g., stereotypically well-dressed, college-educated)	A healthcare professional responds to a patient's request by personally calling a consulting specialist to advocate for the patient, when they would not have done so otherwise

3.3 Bias Among Healthcare Professionals

Although healthcare professionals have the important and laudable goal of providing impartial care, there is no evidence to support that becoming a healthcare professional eliminates one's biases. Rather, healthcare professionals have been shown in multiple studies to have biases similar to the general population [3]. There is no "gold standard" for identification or quantifying biases that an individual may hold. Evidence of bias on the part of healthcare professionals tends to fall into the following categories [3, 4]:

- Implicit bias: Examples include the Implicit Assumption Test (IAT). Healthcare professionals are given this test and compared to other populations, and IAT results are correlated with clinical outcomes.
- Quasi-experimental: Examples include healthcare professionals being given clinical vignettes that differ only in a factor controlled by the investigator and asked about an aspect of care such as attitudes, diagnostic impressions, testing, or treatment.
- Outcomes data: Multiple studies show inequities in outcomes by a patient's race and ethnicity for cardiovascular care, pain management, and transplantation, to name but a few [5]. While some outcome disparities may be caused by complex systems, others are determined at the provider level (e.g., pain medication orders), strongly suggesting individual-level racism or other biases as at least part of the mechanism.

While healthcare professionals as a group may have similar biases to that of the general population, there is variability among individuals.

3.4 Potentially Harmful Language Practices in Medical Chart Notes

Bias, therefore, is a given; but not all bias leads to biased behavior or actions. One action that healthcare professionals take multiple times per day is to document their impressions and activities in the medical record.

3.4.1 Positive and Negative Language

There is evidence that bias can enter into medical notes. Park et al. conducted a qualitative study of outpatient internal medicine chart notes and characterized language use into "positive" and "negative" categories (Tables 3.3 and 3.4) [6].

Negative language may reflect a negative attitude or stance on the part of the note writer toward the patient and should be minimized, if not eliminated completely, in

Table 3.3 Negative language categories

Categories	Definitions	Examples
Questioning credibility	Implication of physician disbelief of patient reports of their own experience or behaviors	• He insists the pain is behind his knee • He claims that nicotine patches don't work for him • I listed several fictitious medication names and she reported she was taking them, and that she takes "whatever is written there"
Disapproval	Highlights poor reasoning, decision-making, or self-care, usually in a way that conveys the patient is unreasonable	• Reports that if she were to fall, she would just "lay there" until someone found her • He was adamant that he does not have prostate cancer because his "bowels are working fine" • Counseled that there is no evidence for this, but patient has strong beliefs • She is adamant that she cannot perform any kind of exercise due to pain and will not change her diet
Stereotyping	Quoting African American Vernacular English	• Chief complaint—"I stay tired"
	Quoting incorrect grammar or unsophisticated terms	• Reports that the bandage got "a li'l wet" • States that the lesion "busted open" • Reports she was unable to fill prescription for the "sugar pill"
Difficult patient	Inclusion of details with questionable clinical significance that depict the patient as belligerent or otherwise suggests that the physician is annoyed	• She perseverated on the fact that "a lot of stuff is going on at home with my family" but that "you wouldn't understand" • I informed her that this is unlikely to be helped by antibiotics and talked about smoking cessation with her. She said she will ask her 'sinus doctor' for antibiotics
Unilateral decisions	Language that emphasizes physician authority over patient	• She was told to discontinue … • I have instructed him to …

From: Park J, Saha S, Chee B, Taylor J, Beach MC. Physician use of stigmatizing language in patient medical records. JAMA Netw Open. 2021;4(7):e2117052. Categories may overlap; examples are from actual chart notes. [Open Access]

favor of more neutral language. Positive language may also be problematic if distributed in a discriminatory fashion—for example, if a provider writes more complimentary statements about patients who are similar in some aspect of identity to the writer.

Rather, the goal is to be thoughtful about what is truly necessary to incorporate in a patient chart and to make sure that what is entered is as unbiased as possible.

Table 3.4 Positive language categories

Categories	Definitions	Examples
Compliment	Explicit adjectives to describe patient positively	• Mr. [Patient] is charming, pleasant, and kind
		• Mrs. [Patient] is a delightful female
Approval	Highlighting patient knowledge, character, reasoning skills, and self-care patient behaviors	• She has a physical/mental robustness that belies her age. She remembers both recent and distant events and is enjoyable to converse with on many subjects
		• She struggled with quitting over the spring and summer but as of this clinic visit has quit tobacco for 1 week!!
		• I provided much deserved praise and encouraged her to continue her trajectory
Self-disclosure	Physician self-disclosure of their own positive emotions related to patient	• I am happy to continue coordinating her care
		• I am also encouraged by his new spirit to improve his health
Minimizing blame	Reports reduced patient capacity or unhealthy behaviors with patient-centered reasons that convey understanding and minimize blame	• She has not been checking her morning glucose for a month because she lost her blood glucose monitor
		• She has not been taking iron because it makes her constipated
Personalize	Incorporation of details about the patient as an individual or particular person	• She is a song writer and also sings. She has a strong faith in God and believes that he has blessed her and continues to keep her strong in light of her progressive disease
		• She enjoys walking with her fiancé and her dog named Scout
Bilateral decision-making	References to the incorporation of patient preferences into the treatment plan	• He does not want to add a medication so I will increase the dose
		• She stated that even if it was positive, she would not want further testing. She will think about this and let me know next time if she wishes to proceed

From: Park J, Saha S, Chee B, Taylor J, Beach MC. Physician use of stigmatizing language in patient medical records. JAMA Netw Open. 2021;4(7):e2117052. Categories may overlap; examples are from actual chart notes. [Open Access]

3.4.2 Labeling

To label a patient is to assign them to a named category. When evaluating a patient, describing their presentation as a series of labels or categories can be helpful in developing a differential diagnosis. For example, a clinician might consider the case of an immune suppressed patient with a fever and a cough differently than that of a person who has an intact immune system. In their mind the provider has labeled the patient (as immune suppressed) in a way that is likely helpful to aid diagnostic reasoning.

Some labels however can lack real medical value, and others can even be harmful to patients:

- Labeling patients as their disease: Most patients prefer to be known as people, not as the disease or condition they may happen to have. For example, calling a patient with diabetes *a diabetic* or a patient with extensive cardiovascular disease a *vasculopath* can have the effect of reducing the patient to their medical condition.
- Labeling patients as *nonadherent* or *noncompliant*: It may be factually true that a patient does not complete a recommendation from their healthcare provider, but these terms tend to effectively label the patient in a negative manner. Especially in the era of the EHR, labels can follow patients indefinitely and can be difficult to unwind.
- Labeling patients as *difficult*: As discussed in Chap. 14, it is better to consider a challenging interaction as difficult, not the patient themselves. As with noncompliance, a label of *difficult* can be hard for a patient to undo once it is in an electronic record and may bias future healthcare interactions irreparably.
- Labeling patients in identifying parts of the note: The identification statement, the first line of the HPI, the first line of the physical exam, and, if used, the summative line at the start of the Assessment and Plan all can be locations where a patient is labeled, either by their medical condition, demographic characteristics, social factors, behavioral characteristics, gender, or other means (Chaps. 7, 12, and 13). The vast majority of labels used in these settings are unnecessary and potentially harmful.

3.4.3 Quotations and Other Language Marking

It is not only words themselves that matter but also how they are written and displayed. For example, even the use of punctuation has evolved: with text messaging the period has evolved from simply closing a sentence to potentially expressing anger or disapproval—this change is not absolute and may yet evolve further. Email has further changed the written language.

For medical notes, the use of quotations can be a signal by their very inclusion. In the study by Park et al. discussed above, the authors identified that when a note writer chooses to directly quote a patient with the use of text within a quotation mark, it can imply doubt or judgment.

> They said that the "flu shot gives me the flu." [expresses doubt]
> They said that they will "go find another doctor." [expresses negative judgment about the patient's ideas or plans]

Quotations have therefore evolved in meaning beyond their original use. This observation however does not mean that quotations are always doubting or judgmental. For example, in the palliative care setting, direct quotes from a patient or family member can often capture the uniqueness and individuality of their wishes:

> ___ expressed their hopes in the following way: "My granddaughter is like the star that shines all night. I just want to see her graduate in June, then I'll be ready to go."

Some specialties such as psychiatry use quotations extensively and appropriately—rather than picking out an occasional phrase or sentence to quote, psychiatrists often record multiple statements verbatim to capture a patient's history more richly. Quotations are often used in the HPI (see Chap. 7). If a quotation is being considered outside of fields in which extensive quotations are used commonly, then it is a best practice to re-read it and to think about one's intentions as well as how it may appear even if the intent is positive.

Other ways a note writer can emphasize text—especially with the EHR—includes variations in font, such as size, italics, and color. These variations have not been extensively studied. For example, an EHR template may automatically change color for positive findings or laboratory values outside the reference interval:

> Review of Systems:
> Constitutional: negative for fevers, chills. Positive for **obesity**.

Emphasis in this manner may lead to a patient feeling being labeled or stigmatized, even if that was not the intention of the note writer.

3.4.4   Evidence that Negative Language Is Distributed Unequally

Beach et al. conducted a study of language that casts doubt on a patient's credibility [7]. The authors analyzed 600 outpatient notes at an academic medical center and grouped doubting language into three categories: evidentials (choosing to indicate the source of information—e.g., writing that a patient *reports* something rather than simply stating the history), judgment words (e.g., *adamant*, *claims*, *insists*), and the use of quotations (when used, can be an indication of doubt as discussed above). They then compared over 9000 notes for the use of these language types between patients identified in the EHR as Black/African American and White/Caucasian. In adjusted analyses, they found that patients who identified as Black/African American had 0.32 more evidentials per note compared to patients who identified as White/Caucasian. Further, judgment words and quotations were more likely to be found in notes of Black/African American compared to White/Caucasian patients, with adjusted odds ratios of 1.25 for judgment words and 1.48 for quotations. In analysis by gender, women were more likely to have quotations used compared to men (odds ratio 1.22), but there was no significant difference in the use of evidentials or judgment words.

Himmelstein et al. conducted a study of inpatient admission notes at an academic medical center [8]. They examined the use of stigmatizing words in notes and found an overall prevalence of 2.5% of notes containing stigmatizing words in a large sample of 48,651 notes. They found that notes of non-Hispanic Black patients were more likely to contain stigmatizing language than those of non-Hispanic White patients (race and ethnicity were extracted from the EHR). These differences were present when analyzed by patients with diabetes, chronic pain, and substance use disorders. Of the potentially stigmatizing words examined, words related to adherence (*nonadherence, adherence, compliance, refused*), perceived attitude (*belligerent, unwilling, difficult patient*), and substance use (*abuse, drug-seeking*) were more strongly associated with a disparity between non-Hispanic Black and non-Hispanic White patients. Patients with diabetes were also found to have an association between disease severity and increased stigmatizing language in their notes.

Sun et al. analyzed patient notes from a dataset of patients tested for COVID-19 at a different academic medical center from Beach et al. and Himmelstein et al. [9]. Their sample included over 18,000 patients who had over 40,000 notes from the outpatient, emergency department, and inpatient settings. They found that 8.2% of patients had at least one negative descriptor (from a list of 15 descriptor categories). Prevalence data is not directly comparable to Himmelstein et al., as they assessed prevalence by patient rather than by note, the stigmatizing words were similar but not exactly the same, and they looked at a wider range of care settings. Similar to Himmelstein et al., the authors found racial disparities in the use of stigmatizing language, with patients who identified as Black based on EHR data having 2.5 times the adjust odds of having negative descriptors compared to patients identified as White.

Limitations of these studies include that they used EHR-based race, ethnicity, and gender data, of which the data collection method was not verified; what words are considered stigmatizing does not have a single consensus; and the natural language processing techniques allow for large volumes of data but cannot contextualize all language use (e.g., quotations are not 100% doubting).

Still, because these studies used natural language processing, with the availability of modern computing power in combination with widespread EHR adoption, it is expected that more studies will be completed to further refine the prevalence and disparities in the use of stigmatizing language across different care settings and regions.

3.5   The Effect of Language on Patients

Is there evidence that negative or stigmatizing language is harmful to patients? Fernandez et al. analyzed a survey of over 20,000 patients across three different health systems and found that, of patients who had read at least one chart note, 10.5% reported feeling judged and/or offended by something they read in the note [10]. Qualitative analysis of free-text responses yielded three themes: Errors and Surprises (e.g., a diagnosis that was not discussed or mistakes in the record or what were perceived as lies), Labeling, and Disrespect (e.g., condescending tone or statements, being misquoted) (Table 3.5). Respondents reported being offended at both positive (e.g., *well-groomed, pleasant, delightful*) and negative descriptors (e.g., *elderly, anxious*).

It is likely that the providers in this study did not experience one in ten patients requesting to speak about language in their chart—based on these results, it is probable that patients react to language in their notes but do not necessarily speak up about it (see Chap. 1).

Table 3.5 Thematic analysis from Fernandez et al. [10] of domains in which patients felt judged or offended reading their chart notes

Theme	Examples
Errors[a]	• Inaccuracy
	• Documentation of something such as a physical exam that was not done
	• Text thought to be an intentional lie
Surprises[a]	• Diagnosis not discussed during the visit
	• Something mentioned to the provider that they thought would not be put in the chart
Disrespect	• Being doubted—words such as *claims, insists*
	• Being misquoted
Labeling	• Obesity mentioned even if not a focus of the visit
	• Descriptors both positive and negative (e.g., *pleasant*, anxious) • Descriptors of general appearance (e.g., *well-groomed*)
	• Substance use
	• Mental health diagnoses
	• Sexuality
	• Gender
	• Age

[a]Errors and Surprises were a single theme in Fernandez et al.; they are separated here for teaching purposes

3.6 The Effect of Language on Diagnosis and Treatment

The study by Fernandez et al. provides evidence that language in written chart notes can directly cause harm to patients. The next question is whether biased language can influence other readers of a chart note. Goddu et al. studied just this question in a quasi-experimental study in which they randomized internal medicine residents, emergency medicine residents, and medical students to read either one of two clinical vignettes, one with neutral language and the other with stigmatizing language [11]. They then asked the residents how much pain medication they would give the patient in the vignette and asked all respondents about their attitudes toward the patient. Residents who received the stigmatizing vignette selected a lower dose of pain medications compared to those who received the neutral vignette (Table 3.6). Subjects who received the neutral vignette had a significantly more positive attitude toward the patient compared to those who received the stigmatizing vignette.

Kelly et al. showed similar findings in mental health professionals given vignettes with the terms *substance abuser* versus *substance use disorder* (see Chap. 10) [12]. Mamede et al. conducted a study of internal medicine residents in Europe, giving them vignettes that were identical except for patient behavior which was either neutral or "difficult," and found that diagnostic accuracy was less in residents who were given the vignette of the "difficult" patient [13]. Although this study was intended to demonstrate changes in diagnostic accuracy when faced with a disruptive patient, because of the vignette-based nature of the study, in which the "difficult" patient vignette used many negative language attributes (e.g., words such as *insists* and the use of quotations), the results may be at least partially due to the effect of negative language in the written vignette. (Also see Chap. 14 for discussion of difficult encounters.) Limitations of such quasi-experimental data are that subjects are asked what they would do, but actual outcomes are not measured. However, it would be unethical to conduct a randomized trial of biased chart notes versus neutral chart notes in a real-world setting. Observational studies also provide useful information but are limited by confounders.

Table 3.6 Quasi-experimental data from Goddu et al. [11] showing the effect of stigmatizing language on provider attitudes and treatment plan

Vignette	Example text	Pain management[a]	Attitude toward patient[b]
Neutral	He is not tolerating the oxygen mask and still has 10/10 pain	5.3	25.5
Stigmatizing	He refuses to wear his oxygen mask and is insisting that his pain is "still a 10"	4.7	20.3

[a]Scale of 2–7; higher scores indicate more pain medication was selected; $p < 0.001$
[b]Scale of 7–35; higher scores represent more positive attitude toward the patient; $p < 0.001$

3.7 Basic Approaches to Improving Language in Chart Notes

Throughout this book we will consider various ways to make language in medical notes and other parts of the EHR less stigmatizing and more patient-centered. The chapters will consider the individual parts of a typical medical note. Table 3.7 shows several general approaches to making language less harmful to patients.

Table 3.7 Basic approaches to making medical charts more patient-centered

Approach	Discussion
Delete/do not include	• Simply not including a potentially harmful word or phrase is often sufficient
	• Will likely not diminish clinical care
	• Will decrease charting time
	• Example: not including race, ethnicity, or language preference in an opening identification statement (see Chap. 7); not including *pleasant* or *cooperative* in the physical exam
Substitute	• Straightforward, generally not more time-intensive
	• Example: *history of substance use disorder* rather than *drug user*
No surprises	• Do not include concerning diagnoses in the note if not discussed in person
Prepare patients for jargon	• Do not use harmful jargon; some jargon however represents appropriate medical terminology and may be retained in notes
	• Explain to patients that they may not understand all the medical terminology in notes they read
	• Be aware of commonly misunderstood (but legitimate) terms such as heart failure, end-stage liver disease; benign conditions that are nevertheless serious; positive findings meaning present, not necessarily good
Prepare patients for confidentiality	• Chart is accessible by members of the patient's healthcare team
	• If a patient would like something not to be included in the chart, they need to explicitly say so and discuss the pros/cons with the provider
Minimize quotations	• Quotations may be used, but re-read to make sure they are being used in a patient-centered manner to better capture the patient's narrative and not in a doubting or condescending way

3.8   Language and Bias: A Framework

The concepts discussed constitute the foundations of a framework to consider how bias infuses language, which can then in turn bias the next reader.

As shown in Fig. 3.1, in a typical healthcare encounter, a patient and healthcare professional ("Note Writer") have a clinical interaction (1), during or after which the note writer documents the encounter (2). The next healthcare professional ("Note Reader") reads the note in preparation for seeing the patient (3) and then interacts with the patient (4). This cycle is repeated as each clinician interacts with the patient and provides documentation. (This framework is simplified as a set of 1:1 encounters for illustrative purposes—there are group dynamics and non-encounter-based interactions such as emails that are not addressed in this framework.)

Figure 3.2 illustrates how bias may affect the interplay between healthcare professionals, the patient, and the written documentation for that patient. In this framework, the same interaction takes place between a patient and a healthcare professional (Note Writer) (1). However, in this case, the clinician writing the note has biases that are infused into the written note (2). While all people have biases, the key feature here is that those biases are reflected in the patient's documentation. The next

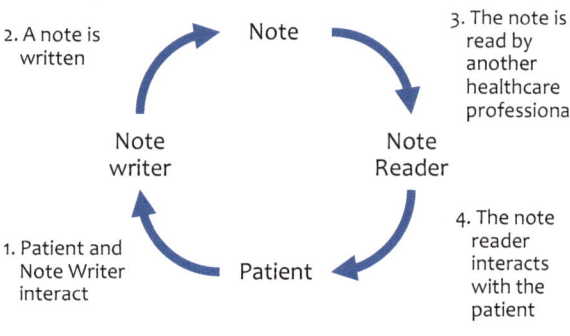

Fig. 3.1 Framework: Relationship between healthcare professionals, the patient, and the patient's documentation

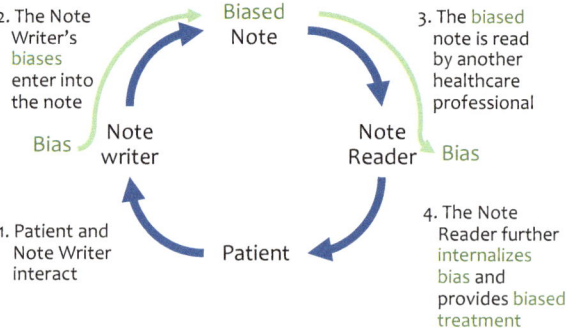

Fig. 3.2 Framework: Bias affects the interaction between healthcare professionals, the patient, and the patient's documentation

healthcare professional reads that note (3) and is at risk for both internalizing those biases, as well as potentially providing biased treatment (positive or negative) to the patient (4).

A goal of this book is to teach healthcare professionals who document clinical encounters to write notes that are more patient-centered—to reduce the creation of a biased note as in the upper left part of Fig. 3.2. Writing about a patient is a deliberate and active process and is susceptible to bias. But because it is an active process, there is potential for improvement with education and training.

Teaching to *write* less biased, more patient-centered notes may not change our actual biases; it is possible however that by being more aware as we document that we may slowly reduce our internal biases, although there is no evidence at this time to support that idea. Further, it is likely that, by being more mindful of one's own note writing, when reading notes authored by other clinicians, one would read with a more critical eye toward recognizing biases within other notes.

3.9 Summary

All people are susceptible to bias toward others, and healthcare professionals are no exception. There is evidence that clinicians may write notes that reflect their own biases toward patients and that the language used in clinical notes may then affect the next clinician who reads the note and lead them toward biased treatment of the patient. While very little research has consistently found a proven intervention to reduce one's own biases, we can pay more careful attention to the way we document in medical charts to reduce the perpetuation and propagation of those biases that we all have.

References

1. Stevenson A, Lindberg CA, editors. New American Oxford Dictionary. Apple Mac Software. Accessed 6 Dec 2022.
2. Zestcott CA, Blair IV, Stone J. Examining the presence, consequences, and reduction of implicit bias in health care: a narrative review. Group Process Intergroup Relat. 2016;19(4):528–42. https://doi.org/10.1177/1368430216642029.
3. FitzGerald C, Hurst S. Implicit bias in healthcare professionals: a systematic review. BMC Med Ethics. 2017;18(1):19. https://doi.org/10.1186/s12910-017-0179-8.
4. Chapman EN, Kaatz A, Carnes M. Physicians and implicit bias: how doctors may unwittingly perpetuate health care disparities. J Gen Intern Med. 2013;28(11):1504–10. https://doi.org/10.1007/s11606-013-2441-1.
5. Institute of Medicine (US) Committee on Understanding and Eliminating Racial and Ethnic Disparities in Health Care. In: Smedley BD, Stith AY, Nelson AR, editors. Unequal treatment: confronting racial and ethnic disparities in health care. Washington, DC: National Academies Press (US); 2003.

6. Park J, Saha S, Chee B, Taylor J, Beach MC. Physician use of stigmatizing language in patient medical records. JAMA Netw Open. 2021;4(7):e2117052. https://doi.org/10.1001/jamanetworkopen.2021.17052.

7. Beach MC, Saha S, Park J, Taylor J, Drew P, Plank E, Cooper LA, Chee B. Testimonial injustice: linguistic bias in the medical records of black patients and women. J Gen Intern Med. 2021;36(6):1708–14. https://doi.org/10.1007/s11606-021-06682-z.

8. Himmelstein G, Bates D, Zhou L. Examination of stigmatizing language in the electronic health record. JAMA Netw Open. 2022;5(1):e2144967. https://doi.org/10.1001/jamanetworkopen.2021.44967.

9. Sun M, Oliwa T, Peek ME, Tung EL. Negative patient descriptors: documenting racial bias in the electronic health record. Health Aff (Millwood). 2022;41(2):203–11. https://doi.org/10.1377/hlthaff.2021.01423.

10. Fernández L, Fossa A, Dong Z, Delbanco T, Elmore J, Fitzgerald P, Harcourt K, Perez J, Walker J, DesRoches C. Words matter: what do patients find judgmental or offensive in outpatient notes? J Gen Intern Med. 2021;36(9):2571–8. https://doi.org/10.1007/s11606-020-06432-7.

11. Goddu AP, O'Conor KJ, Lanzkron S, Saheed MO, Saha S, Peek ME, Haywood C Jr, Beach MC. Do words matter? Stigmatizing language and the transmission of bias in the medical record. J Gen Intern Med. 2018;33(5):685–91. Erratum in: J Gen Intern Med. 2019;34(1):164. https://doi.org/10.1007/s11606-017-4289-2.

12. Kelly JF, Westerhoff CM. Does it matter how we refer to individuals with substance-related conditions? A randomized study of two commonly used terms. Int J Drug Policy. 2010;21(3):202–7. https://doi.org/10.1016/j.drugpo.2009.10.010.

13. Mamede S, Van Gog T, Schuit SC, Van den Berge K, Van Daele PL, Bueving H, Van der Zee T, Van den Broek WW, Van Saase JL, Schmidt HG. Why patients' disruptive behaviours impair diagnostic reasoning: a randomised experiment. BMJ Qual Saf. 2017;26(1):13–8.

Chapter 4
General Principles: Race, Ethnicity, and Gender

Sheida Aalami, Scott Hagan, and Christopher J. Wong

4.1 Introduction

The subjects of race, ethnicity, and gender are areas in which language that is commonly used may be harmful to patients. These topics can be challenging to healthcare professionals as terminology and concepts have evolved over time and likely will continue to evolve. Asking and understanding how patients define themselves and honoring this in written chart notes can enhance patient trust and engagement. In this chapter we discuss patient-centered language issues and offer suggestions for better writing practices.

4.2 Race and Ethnicity

4.2.1 Terminology

While often used synonymously in colloquial speech, race and ethnicity are distinct entities (Table 4.1).

There is no consensus definition of race. Merriam-Webster defines race as "any of the groups that humans are often divided into based on physical traits regarded as common among people of shared ancestry" [1]. Importantly, however, race is a social construct and not a biological one. A better working definition of race is the following: "A socially created and poorly defined categorization of people into groups on basis of real or perceived physical characteristics" [3]. While people with

S. Aalami · S. Hagan · C. J. Wong (✉)
Division of General Internal Medicine, Department of Medicine, University of Washington, Seattle, WA, USA
e-mail: sheida@uw.edu; scotthag@uw.edu; cjwong@uw.edu

© The Author(s), under exclusive license to Springer Nature Switzerland AG 2023
C. J. Wong, S. L. Jackson (eds.), *The Patient-Centered Approach to Medical Note-Writing*, https://doi.org/10.1007/978-3-031-43633-8_4

Table 4.1 Race, ethnicity, and ancestry

Race	"Any of the groups that humans are often divided into based on physical traits regarded as common among people of shared ancestry" [1]
Ethnicity	An affiliation or group "classed according to a common racial, national, tribal, religious, linguistic, or cultural origin or background" [2]
Ancestry	Temporally and geographically, where in the world one's ancestors are thought to have originated from

similar physical traits may share ancestry, they also may not; racial categories are based on arbitrary phenotypic boundaries (such as skin color) and should not be used as a proxy for shared ancestry or shared genetic background.

Ethnicity may be defined as an affiliation or group "classed according to a common racial, national, tribal, religious, linguistic, or cultural origin or background" [2]. Ethnicity, too, is a social construct and does not have a biological basis.

Ancestry: Ancestry may be defined as where in the world a person's ancestors came from. However, given the current consensus of humanity's origins in Africa, people are more commonly interested in ancestry at a closer time point, for historical research (e.g., genealogy research, often on the scale of hundreds of years) or for the study of health (e.g., genetics research, often on the scale of tens of thousands of years, when modern humans were thought to have dispersed from Africa and after which geographic clustering of certain genetic traits may have developed).

Unlike race and ethnicity, ancestry does have a genetic basis for differences between groups of people. However, the science of determining ancestry is itself in evolution. Commercial DNA tests for ancestry are often based on models developed using genomes of present-day people. Such models are still being refined to improve inferences of ancestry based on a present-day individual's DNA. If DNA tests are not available, then a patient's handed-down family ancestry history may be all that is available, and it, too, is not always known with certainty. Because of these limitations with both a patient's family history and commercial DNA testing, one should be cautious with the use of ancestry for clinical decision-making.

Race and ethnicity are sometimes used to make inferences about ancestry. However, while there may be some degree of correlation between either race and ancestry or ethnicity and ancestry in select situations, it is not recommended to make broad generalizations about ancestry based on self-reported race or ethnicity, especially in routine clinical practice. In appropriate settings such as genetic counseling, ethnicity may be one component of a thorough family history that is part of clinical decision-making.

4.2.2 Data Collection

While race is a social construct and not a biological one, we do not advocate ignoring race. Race is inextricably tied to numerous health outcomes not through biology, but through the social experience of race. In the United States, for example, Black and indigenous people are at a higher risk of poor health outcomes [4] related to the enslavement of Black people, the genocide of indigenous communities, and the ongoing legacies of racism, discrimination, the differential treatment, and related chronic stress that followed.

Generally, patients think it is important they are asked about their racial and ethnic identities but also concerned with how this information may be used to discriminate against them [5]. We recommend that data on patients' self-identified race and ethnicity be collected at registration with other demographic information. This data collection should be systematic to reduce bias (Table 4.2). Multiple racial and ethnic categories should be included, including an "other" category with a write-in option for patients whose specific racial and ethnic identities do not fit the preselected categories.

Health systems should take great care not to solely include the 1997 United States Office of Management and Budget racial and ethnic categories, which were intended to be a minimum, and leave behind much of the population. Racial categories set by the government have changed over time, often every 10 years with each census in the United States, supporting that they are fluid social constructs rather than biologic in nature [6]. Patients should also be given the opportunity to decline to answer without real or perceived repercussions. Declining to answer, not knowing, and simply leaving the question blank are not the same and should not be conflated. Systematic data collection through the EHR is important as it allows the EHR to be used as a tool for quality improvement interventions to reduce racial

Table 4.2 Data collection recommendations for race and ethnicity

Registration	• Use a systematic method of collecting data, e.g., registration staff who are trained in asking patients about identity
	• Provide multiple methods of collecting data: in-person, EHR portal, paper forms
	• Language services
	• Disability accessibility
Purpose	• Purpose stated clearly (e.g., quality improvement, required governmental regulations)
Patient education	• Clearly state that both race and ethnicity are social constructs. Asking about race and ethnicity is not meant to imply that they are biological
Setting	• Include as part of demographic or social history (not as part of medical conditions)
Choices	• Offer a wide range of possible races and ethnicities
	• Do not include multiple options in a single selection (e.g., "Hispanic/Latino/Latina/Latinx," "Native Hawaiian or Pacific Islander," "Don't know/decline to answer")
	• Allow selecting multiple options
	• Include a write-in option
	• Include a "decline to answer" option
	• Allow patients to not select any options (i.e., patient is not forced to answer before moving on to the next question if entering online)

disparities. Ancestry data is not commonly collected but is an area of future EHR development.

4.2.3 Race and Ethnicity: How Should They Be Represented in the Medical Note?

Since race and ethnicity are both social and not biological constructs, they should only be included in chart notes within that context (e.g., Social History) (Table 4.3).

Although it has been historically taught and is still commonly done [7, 8], race and ethnicity should generally not be included in "one-liners," such as the Identification/Reason for Visit, or the first line of the History of Present Illness (HPI) (see Chap. 7). Including race in the opening description incorrectly presents race as a biomedical concept and serves to bias the reader upfront by labeling the patient at the very start of the note. For the vast majority of the reasons for presentation, race is not relevant and certainly not paramount enough to be elevated to the opening statement. Even if such information were valid to include, it is unlikely that busy clinicians take an accurate racial and ethnic history on every patient for every encounter or verify EHR data if racial and ethnic data is present.

Sometimes patients will share experiences of racism within and outside of the healthcare system. They may share prior negative interactions or experiences and feelings of differential treatment due to their race. These discussions should be

Table 4.3 Race and ethnicity in medical notes

Location	• Part of Social History if history is obtained appropriately
	• Should generally not be included in "one-liners" either as the identification statement, the first line of the HPI
	• Should not be included as an examination finding
Discussion	• If race and ethnicity are discussed as a risk factor for conditions or treatment outcomes, they should not be assumed to be based on biologic differences, but rather:
	– They may have a genetic basis only *if* they do correlate with ancestry
	– They may have a basis in social factors such as discrimination
	• Race and ethnicity should not be assumed to be a proxy for ancestry
	• Ancestry—if can be determined—may change the likelihood of certain genes being present
Risk of biased notes based on racial or ethnic stereotypes	• Stigmatizing language in medical notes is not distributed evenly among racial groups
	• Less biased note-writing practices are recommended, even if they do not necessarily change one's own biases

documented similarly to other patient concerns and, depending on the context, may be appropriate for the HPI or the Social History (see Chap. 9).

Because race is a social construct and not an objective finding, it should never be included in physical exam section (Chap. 12). If it is clinically important to describe skin color (e.g., to stratify skin cancer risk), then it is better to use a more objective scale such as the Fitzpatrick scale, although it too remains an imperfect tool to classify skin pigment [9].

A good racial and ethnic history can be part of a patient's holistic social history. If being asked via interview, race and ethnicity should be asked via open-ended questions and should be just one part of a patient's identity that may encompass other identities including gender, profession, family, and other societal roles. While this book does not specifically address the medical interview, an example invitation to address these topics is the following: "Some patients have racial, ethnic, gender, religious or other identities they feel are important that their health care team know about. Is there anything you would like to share with me to help me understand who you are as a person?"

4.2.4 Race and Ethnicity in Medical Notes: Biological Concepts

Inappropriate biological concepts of race have permeated medicine [10]. As such, these racialized elements are often incorporated, whether intentionally or not, into medical notes.

One example is in the use of clinical algorithms or estimation tools that include race or ethnicity as predictive variables. An equation for estimating kidney function that includes race as a modifier has been challenged and is increasingly no longer accepted [11, 12]. Other clinical algorithms that used race or ethnicity as a variable include measures of lung function [6] and risk of cardiovascular events [13]. If these data elements are in medical documentation, providers may need to explain to patients the limitations and controversies surrounding the use of race within formulas.

Providers may also harbor their own view of biological differences between races and ethnicities, and their notes may reflect those beliefs; patients reading such notes may appropriately challenge such statements.

4.2.5 Racial Bias in Medical Notes

Racial bias can take many forms in medical documentation. There is evidence that the stigmatizing language discussed in Chap. 3 and elsewhere in this book varies by many factors, one of which is a patient's race (in most studies, race is identified from demographic EHR data). In a study of outpatient clinic notes, providers more frequently used doubting language (e.g., use of quotations and words such as *claims* and *insists*) in notes of patients who were identified in chart demographics as Black or African-American [14]. Similarly, a natural language study of admission notes found that patients identified as non-Hispanic Black had higher rates of stigmatizing language compared to those identified as non-Hispanic White [15]. Another natural language study of inpatient, outpatient, and emergency department notes at a different center found that patients who identified as Black based on EHR data had 2.5 times the adjusted odds of having negative descriptors (e.g., *refused* or *(not) compliant*) compared to patients identified as White [16].

4.3 Gender

4.3.1 Terminology

For such a commonly used term, it may come as a surprise that there is no consensus definition of gender [17].

The following terms are definitions that will be used in this book (Table 4.4). We recognize that nomenclature will likely evolve over time toward terms with greater precision and increased consensus. It should also be recognized that patients may prefer one set of terms over another.

- Sex: Categories typically include Male, Female, and Intersex. Sex generally refers to either a person's chromosomal arrangement (e.g., XX for female, XY for male) or phenotypic appearance at birth with respect to reproductive organs. However, these terms are generally inadequate for situations in which there is sex gender ambiguity based on phenotype or organs, other chromosomal variations, and sex hormone resistance syndromes in which the phenotype does not correspond to the expected phenotype based on chromosomal arrangement.
- Gender: Categories may include male, female, nonbinary, and gender nonconforming. Gender refers to a person's self-identification as a member one of the gender identity classes. This usage is synonymous with gender identity and is distinct from sex. However, some people use the term gender interchangeably with sex.
- Cisgender: The state of having a gender identity that the same as the sex that was assigned at birth.
- Transgender: The state of having a gender identity that is different than the sex that was assigned at birth.
- Assigned (sex) at birth: The sex assigned to a person at birth. Terms may include Assigned Female At Birth (sometimes abbreviated as AFAB) and Assigned Male At Birth (sometimes abbreviated as AMAB).
- Gender expression: The manner in which a person communicates their gender.

Table 4.4 Gender terminology. The following are working definitions used in this book; there exists variation in uptake and usage

Term	Category examples[a]	Definition	Comment

Sex	• Male
	• Female
	• Intersex
		Either:
		• A person's chromosomal arrangement (e.g., XX for female, XY for male)
		Or:
		• A person's phenotypic appearance at birth with respect to reproductive organs
			• These terms may insufficiently describe situations such as disorders of sex development including:
			  – Sex gender ambiguity based on phenotype or organs
			  – Chromosomal arrangements other than XX or XY
			  – Sex hormone resistance syndromes in which the reproductive organ phenotype does not correspond to the expected phenotype based on chromosomal arrangement
			• In nonmedical use, some use this term synonymously with gender
			• Some refer to "sex gender"

Gender	• Male/Man • Female/Woman • Nonbinary • Gender non-conforming • Gender fluid • Agender • Gender incongruent • Genderqueer	A person's self-identification as a member of a gender identity class	• This usage is distinct from sex • Some use the term gender identity • In nonmedical settings, some use gender interchangeably with sex
Cisgender	N/A	Having a gender identity that is the same as the sex that was assigned at birth	
Transgender	N/A	Having a gender identity that is different than the sex that was assigned at birth	• Transgender is often used as an umbrella term for all genders other than cisgender • However, not all individuals who are not cisgender use this term for themselves

(continued)

Table 4.4 (continued)

Term	Category examples[a]	Definition	Comment
Assigned (sex) at birth	• Assigned Female At Birth (AFAB) • Assigned Male At Birth (AMAB)	The sex assigned to a person at birth	
Gender expression	• Feminine • Masculine • Other	Expression or display of gender	May be different from gender identity

Adapted from UCSF Transgender Care guidelines [18] and Palmer et al. [17]
[a]Examples are not comprehensive, as newer terms are expected to evolve and find use

Having clear terminology is useful for descriptive purposes and classification. Keep in mind, however, that an individual person's identity may not fall precisely into one of these categories. Additionally, one should avoid using the phrase "preferred gender" or in general refer to gender as a preference when referring to a patient's gender identity. A person's gender identity is generally considered not a choice, but rather an innate and internal sense of how they view their gender. However, a patient may have preferences in how they wish to be addressed (i.e., what terms to use) with respect to their gender identity.

For example, a person who was assigned female sex at birth, has XX chromosomes, has typical female reproductive anatomy, and has a female gender identity could be described as Assigned Female At Birth, Cisgender, and Female; she may however identify as Female and prefer only that term. Similarly, a person who is Assigned Male At Birth, has XY chromosomes, had typical male reproductive anatomy at birth, and has a female gender identity may refer to themselves as Transgender, Assigned Male at Birth, and Female; or as a Transwoman or Transgender Woman; or simply prefer Female or Woman without any other descriptors unless discussing gender topically (Table 4.5).

4.3.2   Gender: Data Collection

Ideally, a thorough, systematic, and patient-centered gender history should be obtained for every patient. Table 4.6 shows best practices for data collection. At a minimum, the patient's gender identity and pronouns should be ascertained. This information could be obtained at registration by administrative staff. In general, medical providers should have a variety of means to obtain this type of information, as resources and patient barriers vary. For example, some practice settings may have limited administrative/registration staff or may not have the training for them to obtain gender information in a gender-affirming manner. In other settings, patients may complete forms on their own—however, some patients have less direct access to the EHR for direct entry, and language proficiency and visual impairment may limit the use of paper forms.

Table 4.5 Gender examples[a]

Assigned sex at birth	Cis- or transgender	Chromosome arrangement	Reproductive anatomy	Gender (or gender identity)
Female	Cis	XX	Female	Female or Woman
Male	Cis	XY	Male	Male or Man
Male	Trans	XY	Male	Female or Woman
Male	Trans	XY	Male at birth, now status post-gender-affirming surgery	Female or Woman
Female	Trans	XX	Female	Male or Man
Female	Trans	XX	Female at birth, now status post-gender-affirming surgery	Male or Man
Male	Trans[b]	XY	Male	Nonbinary
Female	Trans[b]	XX	Female	Nonbinary

[a]These examples do not encompass the complete range of gender possibilities but are meant as examples for illustrative purposes
[b]People of nonbinary gender may identify as transgender, as their gender is something other than that assigned at birth; however, not all people with nonbinary gender identify with the term transgender

Table 4.6 Gender data collection: best practices [19]

• Collect name, gender, and pronoun data at registration alongside other demographic information
• Data collection should be systematic (i.e., for all patients) to reduce bias
• Data collection should have multiple methods (in-person, paper forms, EHR forms) as patients may have barriers to a single method
• Language interpretation should be available
• A clinician may also enter data together with the patient or verify data already entered
• Have multiple choices available:
– Do not use only "male," "female," and "other"
– Instead use a wide range of choices including, but not limited to: "male," "female," "nonbinary," "transman," "transwoman," "transgender male," and "transgender female"
– Do not include multiple terms in a single selection
– Include a write-in option
– Allow choice not to disclose
• Allow recognition if data has not been collected adequately (default to "missing" or "not addressed")

Adapted from Grasso et al. [19] and HRSA guidelines [20]

However, there are several reasons why the ideal is often not achieved. As noted above, there may be barriers to systematic collection of information. Additionally, while systematic collection of information reduces bias, that information may need to be verified by the clinician. A patient may have been in a non-gender-affirming environment and may wish to further explore gender identity with their provider before declaring the gender identity into the EHR. Clinicians should also be aware that for some aspects of gender identity and history, patients may not want to reveal them to medical staff whom they do not know well or who may not be making care decisions with them. For example, a transgender patient may provide their gender and pronouns to a front desk staff member, but may not want to discuss details of their anatomy or hormonal care. Nevertheless, this information will need to be obtained for certain important clinical care, such as insurance covering screening related to reproductive organs (e.g., a transgender man may have a cervix and therefore be eligible for cervical cancer screening) [21].

In addition to potential systems barriers to obtaining an accurate gender identity history, there may be challenges to the timing of updating EHR data regarding gender identity or catching up a large number of patients who may already be part of a practice but for whom gender identity was not obtained systematically before. While ideally gender identity should be updated yearly [19], the question is in what setting this would occur. Patients could have updated registration information delivered to them each year, with the same potential barriers as above (e.g., in person, on paper forms, directly into the EHR). Updates by the clinician would typically be done during an annual ("preventive health") visit, as it may be neither appropriate nor feasible during acute care or chronic disease management visits due to competing demands. However, patients do not always receive preventive visits, so clinics may need to find other ways to update this information. Grasso et al. provide guidelines for the implementation of gender identity as well as sexual orientation data collection in clinical practices [19].

4.3.3 Gender: How Should It Be Presented in the EHR?

Data collection and presentation are different aspects of gender-affirming and patient-centered language. Once the data are collected, there are many options and not necessarily one single best way to document a patient's gender in the EHR for all situations.

We suggest the following approach (Table 4.7):

The one-liner or any opening descriptor: The so-called "one-liner" is often an **Identification** or **Chief Concern** (or "chief complaint"—see Chap. 7 regarding discussion of language in these statements) statement at the beginning of a note. Additionally, there is typically a descriptive statement as the first line of the History of Present Illness and sometimes a summary description at the beginning of the Assessment and Plan (see Chap. 13).

- Include the patient's gender identity (example: male/man, female/woman, non-binary person) after their age if the gender identity has been accurately obtained.
- Do not include information such as transgender or cisgender status unless the patient prefers that to be included [22].
- Do not include sex assigned at birth [22].
- Do not use address titles (Mr./Mrs./Ms.) unless verified with the patient.

Table 4.7 Suggested documentation of gender in medical notes

Example	Comment
50-year-old woman here for evaluation of a finger injury 50-year-old man here for follow-up of diabetes 50-year-old nonbinary patient here for follow-up of hypertension	These statements do include gender, but do not make any mention of sex assigned at birth, chromosomes, reproductive anatomy, or cis- or transgender status, as it is likely not relevant to this clinical concern
ID: 50-year-old female here for evaluation of lower abdominal pain HPI: The patient developed abdominal pain in the RLQ 3 days ago, described as sharp, colicky, unrelated to oral intake. She has normal bowel movements. She has no fever, nausea, or vomiting and no prior episodes of similar symptoms She was assigned male at birth and identifies as female; she has male reproductive organs including bilateral testes and penis and has not undergone surgery. She is treated with estrogen for gender-affirming care for the last 10 years	This history does not call out the patient's transgender status in the opening line, but because it is relevant to the evaluation of lower abdominal pain, the patient's anatomy and hormonal treatment are discussed later in the HPI

The History of Present Illness: Here it may be appropriate to include other information obtained about gender.

- Include other gender-related information later in the History of Present Illness if it is relevant. For example, understanding a patient's reproductive organ anatomy is important for the evaluation of lower abdominal or pelvic region pain. Knowing the hormonal history is important when considering risk of pulmonary embolism in a patient presenting with dyspnea.
- Do not assume a gender-related history is relevant. For example, although mental health disorders and a history of trauma are common in transgender people [23, 24], it should not be assumed that a transgender person's mood disorder is related to their gender identity. The history should be explored carefully with the patient to determine its relevance.

Other authors favor different approaches. Some writers favor not putting gender at all in the opening line of a note or presentation, but rather maintaining neutral terms for all patients:

45-year-old person here for follow up of diabetes.

Neutral terms may be particularly useful in form letters or other communications or statements that are not as individualized as a clinical patient encounter. For example, a letter may be written as "Dear Patient" to avoid the issue of a gendered pronoun entirely. (See below for further discussion of gender affirming language.)

Some writers favor the opposite approach by including cis- or transgender status for all patients:

45-year-old cisgender female here for follow up of diabetes

45-year-old transgender male here for follow up of diabetes

If additional terms are used, then they should be used for all patients. For example, one should not document a patient as transgender while not documenting other patients as cisgender, as it would imply cisgender is the normative default.

There are advantages and disadvantages to these various approaches, and there may be an evolution in the consensus manner in which gender is documented in medical notes in the future.

The clinician must be careful to check assumptions. In some cases, patients may be in the process of transitioning their gender expression and may not want to change how their gender is listed in the medical chart or the pronouns. For example, a clinician may be aware that their patient was assigned female at birth and has a gender identity of male, but before changing documented pronouns to he/him and descriptor to male, it is best to check with the patient, as others will also be reading the same medical chart. As with data collection above, a patient's pronouns should be reviewed with them and entered into the EHR as appropriate. And, as noted above, a patient may have different preferences with regard to terms—for example, some transgender patients prefer to be documented as a transwoman or transman, or a transgender male or female, while others may prefer that their medical notes simply list their gender identity without notation of transgender status upfront.

In addition to the clinician's notes, the other logistic decision is how and where that data is stored in a patient's medical chart. Many EHRs now allow the patient to have a gender identity entered into the system such that the appropriate terms will be used in automatic templating (see Chap. 6). We suggest only using templated pronouns in medical notes if that information is reliably and accurately obtained; otherwise, it would be better for a clinician to directly enter the correct pronouns into the note without templating. The gender information itself could "live" in its own section, or in the social history, or in the medical history; the concept of gender may overlap with several parts of the medical chart. In addition, many charts use the term "problem list," but that term can be itself problematic—while clinicians may view it neutrally, gender identity itself is not necessarily a "problem" for a patient (see Chap. 8).

This book focuses on clinical notes; a related issue not covered in depth here is how the data entry for a patient's reproductive organs affects EHR reference ranges and clinical alerts [25]; these are important implementation considerations and may also enter into patient clinical notes if data or reminder elements are imported into those notes.

In addition to the clinician's notes, diagnosis codes include language that may be problematic with respect to gender. For example, entering a transgender history into the problem list or medical history often requires an International Classification of Diseases, 10th Revision (ICD-10) code. Unfortunately, with existing codes that refer to mental health disorders such as Gender Identity Disorder or Gender Dysphoria [17], the patient's gender becomes labeled a disease state, and not all patients who are transgender suffer from a disorder. The same issue applies when assigning a diagnosis code to a clinical encounter, or a medication, or a referral for surgery. Until charting develops more sophisticated tools and/or the next ICD revision improves upon these terms, we suggest that charts avoid the use of terms such as Gender Identity Disorder [22]. If such terms must be used, then the clinician and patient should discuss together the dilemma and arrive at a decision as how to balance potentially stigmatizing or inaccurate coding with the need to have treatment covered. In some cases, alternate codes may be preferred, such as E34.9 (Endocrine Disorder). Some EHRs allow alternative display names for ICD codes (see Chap. 6).

4.3.4 Consequences of Inaccurate and Non-Patient-Centered Gender Language

Having patient-centered language is a worthy goal in and of itself. Additionally, language that is not patient-centered may be harmful to patients and to the patient-clinician relationship. A qualitative study of transgender patients reading their chart notes found that misgendered chart notes caused shame, disappointment, and reduced trust [22]. Further, patients found that chart notes often used quotes when speaking about gender, suggesting doubt on the part of the writer (see Chap. 3 re: use of quotations). These patients further reported stigma at mental health diagnoses being linked to transgender status in one-line summaries and felt that they were inappropriately labeled in one-liners with often unnecessary or inaccurate terms such as FTM (Female-To-Male) or MTF (Male-To-Female).

4.3.5 Gender-Affirming Language and the Use of Neutral Terms

In addition to the above regarding a patient's gender identity, the principles of using gender-affirming language can be applied to other aspects of language in clinical care.

For example, it is generally feasible to avoid gendered terms completely in many situations (Table 4.8). English does not have gendered nouns, but it does have gendered terms. One may refer to a patient as having a *spouse* rather than writing *husband* or *wife* or to use *partner* rather than *boyfriend* or *girlfriend*. (Although we are focusing on written documentation, these concepts apply to verbal communication as well.)

In patient communications such as letters and electronic messages, consider the use of *Dear Patient* or *Dear [first name] [last name]* rather than using a gendered pronoun such as *Mr./Mrs./Ms*. This approach may be especially useful for templated, batch communications in which the communication is not individualized based on knowledge of the patient.

Table 4.8 Suggestions for removing gendered terms in medical documentation and communication

Gendered term	Neutral term
Dear Mr./Mrs./Ms.	Dear Patient
	Dear [First Name + Last Name]
Husband/wife	Spouse
Boyfriend/girlfriend	Partner
Alumni/alumna	Alum
Actor/actress	Actor (for all genders)

If a patient uses a gendered term (e.g., refers to their spouse as *wife* or *husband*), then it is appropriate in a clinical encounter to use that term.

The English language continues to evolve; one of these evolutions is the use of *they* as a singular pronoun for all people, a convention we are using for examples in this book (other than when specifically discussing gender and pronouns; also see Chap. 1 for conventions used in this book), and which is supported by the American Psychological Association style guidelines as well as Merriam-Webster's Dictionary [26]. Some advocate for newer words such as ze/zir; it is uncertain over time which terms will become standard.

Languages other than English vary widely in gendered words—for example, some languages have gendered nouns (e.g., Latin, German, French), while others do not have he/she pronouns at all (e.g., Chinese).

4.3.6 Gender: Biased Language Based on Gender Stereotypes

Gender bias exists in the medical field as it does elsewhere. For example, a quasi-experimental study found that physicians who were presented video vignettes with accompanying data had differential recommendations for cardiac catheterization depending on the patient's race and gender [27].

There is evidence that gender bias is infused into medical note-writing as well. A natural language processing study of 1.8 million ICU notes at an academic medical center over 10 years found that male patients were more likely to have positive emotional terms (examples: *brave*, *success*) and less likely to have negative emotion terms (examples: *bad*, *sick*) [28]. Another study found that notes of female patients were more likely to contain quotations, which in many contexts are used as expressions of doubt about a patient's reported history (see Chaps. 3 and 7) [14]. In contrast, a study of inpatient admission notes did not find a gender difference in the use of stigmatizing language [15].

As with racism and discrimination based on ethnicity, reducing gender-biased language in medical notes may not reduce a person's individual biases, but there is inherent value in recognizing biased language and working to eliminate it as much as possible.

4.4 Conclusion

Race, ethnicity, and gender may be important aspects to a patient's identity. An accurate and appropriately collected history of these elements can add to a holistic view of a patient as an individual. Unfortunately, race, ethnicity, and gender are also sources of bias and discrimination in healthcare, for which those who write in the medical chart are also responsible. With education in up-to-date terminology and patient-centered language practices, healthcare professionals can write notes that foster trust with and earn respect from their patients.

References

1. Merriam-Webster Dictionary. https://www.merriam-webster.com/dictionary/race. Accessed 12 Mar 2023.
2. Merriam-Webster Dictionary. https://www.merriam-webster.com/dictionary/ethnicity, https://www.merriam-webster.com/dictionary/ethnic. Accessed 12 Mar 2023.
3. Open Education Sociology Dictionary. https://sociologydictionary.org/race/. Accessed 12 Mar 2023.
4. Institute of Medicine. Unequal treatment: confronting racial and ethnic disparities in health care. Washington, DC: The National Academies Press; 2003. https://doi.org/10.17226/12875.
5. Baker DW, Cameron KA, Feinglass J, et al. Patients' attitudes toward health care providers collecting information about their race and ethnicity. J Gen Intern Med. 2005;20:895–900.
6. Braun L, Wolfgang M, Dickersin K. Defining race/ethnicity and explaining difference in research studies on lung function. Eur Respir J. 2013;41:1362–70.
7. Nawaz H, Brett AS. Mentioning race at the beginning of clinical case presentations: a survey of US medical schools. Med Educ. 2009;43(2):146–54. https://doi.org/10.1111/j.1365-2923.2008.03257.x.
8. Acquaviva KD, Mintz M. Perspective: are we teaching racial profiling? The dangers of subjective determinations of race and ethnicity in case presentations. Acad Med. 2010;85(4):702–5. https://doi.org/10.1097/ACM.0b013e3181d296c7.
9. Sharma AN, Patel BC. Laser Fitzpatrick skin type recommendations. In: StatPearls. Treasure Island, FL: StatPearls Publishing; 2022. https://www.ncbi.nlm.nih.gov/books/NBK557626/. Accessed 12 Mar 2023.
10. Root M. The problem of race in medicine. Philos Soc Sci. 2000;8(31):20–39.
11. Eneanya ND, Yang W, Reese PP. Reconsidering the consequences of using race to estimate kidney function. JAMA. 2019;322:113–4.
12. Grubbs V. Precision in GFR reporting: let's stop playing the race card. CJASN. 2020;15(8):1201–2. https://doi.org/10.2215/CJN.00690120.
13. Vyas DA, James A, Kormos W, Essien UR. Revising the atherosclerotic cardiovascular disease calculator without race. Lancet Digit Health. 2022;4(1):e4–5. https://doi.org/10.1016/S2589-7500(21)00258-2.
14. Beach MC, Saha S, Park J, Taylor J, Drew P, Plank E, Cooper LA, Chee B. Testimonial injustice: linguistic bias in the medical records of black patients and women. J Gen Intern Med. 2021;36(6):1708–14. https://doi.org/10.1007/s11606-021-06682-z.
15. Himmelstein G, Bates D, Zhou L. Examination of stigmatizing language in the electronic health record. JAMA Netw Open. 2022;5(1):e2144967. https://doi.org/10.1001/jamanetworkopen.2021.44967.

16. Sun M, Oliwa T, Peek ME, Tung EL. Negative patient descriptors: documenting racial bias in the electronic health record. Health Aff (Millwood). 2022;41(2):203–11. https://doi. org/10.1377/hlthaff.2021.01423.

17. Palmer BF, Clegg DJ. A universally accepted definition of gender will positively impact societal understanding, acceptance, and appropriateness of health care. Mayo Clin Proc. 2020;95(10):2235–43. https://doi.org/10.1016/j.mayocp.2020.01.031.

18. UCSF Transgender Care. Terminology and definitions. 17 June 2016. https://transcare.ucsf. edu/guidelines/terminology. Accessed 7 Jan 2023.

19. Grasso C, McDowell MJ, Goldhammer H, Keuroghlian AS. Planning and implementing sexual orientation and gender identity data collection in electronic health records. J Am Med Inform Assoc. 2019;26(1):66–70. https://doi.org/10.1093/jamia/ocy137.

20. Health Resources and Services Administration. Uniform data system: reporting instructions for 2017 health center data. Rockville, MD: Bureau of Primary Healthcare. https://bphc.hrsa. gov/sites/default/files/bphc/data-reporting/2017-uds-reporting-manual.pdf.

21. Goldhammer H, Malina S, Keuroghlian AS. Communicating with patients who have nonbinary gender identities. Ann Fam Med. 2018;16(6):559–62. https://doi.org/10.1370/afm.2321.

22. Alpert AB, Mehringer JE, Orta SJ, Redwood E, Hernandez T, Rivers L, Manzano C, Ruddick R, Adams S, Cerulli C, Operario D, Griggs JJ. Experiences of transgender people reviewing their electronic health records, a qualitative study. J Gen Intern Med. 2023;38(4):970–97. https://doi.org/10.1007/s11606-022-07671-6.

23. Valentine SE, Shipherd JC. A systematic review of social stress and mental health among transgender and gender non-conforming people in the United States. Clin Psychol Rev. 2018;66:24–38. https://doi.org/10.1016/j.cpr.2018.03.003.

24. White BP, Fontenot HB. Transgender and non-conforming persons' mental healthcare experiences: an integrative review. Arch Psychiatr Nurs. 2019;33(2):203–10. https://doi. org/10.1016/j.apnu.2019.01.005.

25. Chittalia AZ, Marney HL, Tavares S, Warsame L, Breese AW, Fisher DL, Stoppie ME, Coen D, Zikowski KA, Shapiro AW, Vawdrey DK. Bringing cultural competency to the EHR: lessons learned providing respectful, quality care to the LGBTQ community. AMIA Annu Symp Proc. 2021;2020:303–10.

26. American Psychological Association. Singular they. Updated July 2022, created September 2019. https://apastyle.apa.org/style-grammar-guidelines/grammar/singular-they. Accessed 14 Jan 2023.

27. Schulman KA, Berline JA, Harless W, Kerner JF, Sistrunk S, Gersh BJ, et al. The effect of race and sex on physicians' recommendations for cardiac catheterization. N Engl J Med. 1999;340:618–26. https://doi.org/10.1056/NEJM199902253400806.

28. Markowitz DM. Gender and ethnicity bias in medicine: a text analysis of 1.8 million critical care records. PNAS Nexus. 2022;1(4):pgac157. https://doi.org/10.1093/pnasnexus/pgac157.

Chapter 5
General Principles: Body Habitus and What Is "Normal"

Scott Hagan, Sheida Aalami, and Christopher J. Wong

5.1 Body Habitus

5.1.1 Clinical Importance of Body Habitus

The body habitus, or the shape and size of the body or body parts of an individual, may have important clinical implications. Both low body mass index (BMI) (less than 18.5 kg/m^2) and high BMI (above 35 kg/m^2) are associated with an increased mortality risk for varying health conditions [1]. Further, independent of total adiposity levels as estimated by BMI, markers of central adiposity, such as waist-to-hip ratio and waist-to-height ratio, are also associated with increased mortality [2]. Finally, the risk of some diseases is elevated when certain parts of the body are larger, such as a neck circumference above 40 cm and the risk for obstructive sleep apnea [3] and the risk for intertrigo in individuals with increased BMI [4].

Separate from adiposity, muscle mass is an important component of the assessment of diseases such as cachexia [5] and the evaluation of muscle weakness [6]. The presence of a high or a low muscle mass is also a criterion for confirmation of creatinine-based estimated GFR with tests such as cystatin C [7]. Therefore, there are many situations in which the accurate description of body habitus in a clinical note may add useful objective information to inform an assessment and plan.

S. Hagan (✉) · S. Aalami · C. J. Wong
Division of General Internal Medicine, Department of Medicine, University of Washington, Seattle, WA, USA
e-mail: scotthag@uw.edu; sheida@uw.edu; cjwong@uw.edu

© The Author(s), under exclusive license to Springer Nature Switzerland AG 2023

C. J. Wong, S. L. Jackson (eds.), *The Patient-Centered Approach to Medical Note-Writing*, https://doi.org/10.1007/978-3-031-43633-8_5

5.1.2 Bias and Stigma in Description of Body Habitus

The description of body habitus in clinical notes is fraught with opportunities to convey the bias of the note's author and to create the perception of discrimination toward the patient. Implicit and explicit anti-fat bias is common among healthcare professionals [8], and in one study, doctors were second only to family members in sources of weight stigma [9]. It is thus unsurprising that patients perceive negative labeling of their body habitus in clinical notes. In one survey, patients commonly felt judged by the documentation of elevated body weight [10], especially when they did not recall a discussion of this topic during the encounter.

5.1.3 Systemic Coding Biases in Description of Body Habitus

A number of International Classification of Diseases (ICD)-10 codes currently include language that is potentially stigmatizing (Table 5.1) [11]. Unfortunately, there are incentives for providers in the Medicare system in the United States to use the code E66.01 (morbid [severe] obesity due to excess calories) as part of the Hierarchical Condition Category (HCC) system of risk adjustment, which confers a high risk to that code, but not to the less stigmatizing codes E66.9 or E66.8. If a provider concludes that using a potentially stigmatizing code should be used for the overall benefit of the patient (e.g., for approval of a treatment), then it is recommended that they discuss with the patient the rationale to use stigmatizing language but also explain that they do not agree with such terms. The language in future iterations of the US version of ICD-10 (and ICD-11 which will be likely be implemented in the United States by 2026) is subject to a periodic review process by the Centers for Disease Control and Prevention, which may change the problematic language (e.g., "morbid," "due to excess calories") in this coding family.

Table 5.1 ICD-10 codes related to weight

Potentially stigmatizing ICD-10 codes	Preferred coding
E66.01: Morbid (severe) obesity due to excess calories	Use a combination of non-stigmatizing obesity code with BMI code:
E66.09: Other obesity due to excess calories	E66.8: Other obesity
E66.2: Morbid (severe) obesity with alveolar hypoventilation	E66.9: Obesity, unspecified
E66.3: Overweight	+
	Z68: Body mass index coding family
	e.g., Z68.35 body mass index [BMI] 35.0–35.9

5.1.4 Patient Preferences Regarding Weight Terms

Many studies have aimed to study patient preferences for language in clinical encounters related to elevated body weight [12]. The survey tool most often used is the Weight Preferences Questionnaire, which provides a prompt to the patient or family member of a hypothetical scenario in which they present to the doctor's office, are found to have an elevated body weight, and are asked what, in a list of terms, they would find desirable or undesirable for a doctor to use to describe their weight [13]. Consistently in this research, patients describe the least favored terminology to be "fat," "obese," and "obesity." Suggestions for alternative terminology in the description of body habitus, both for individuals with a high BMI and for those with a low BMI, are provided in Table 5.2.

Table 5.2 Body habitus terminology: common descriptions and suggested alternatives

Common descriptions of body habitus	Suggested alternative with explanation
Severely obese 50-year-old man	• Use patient-first language when describing an individual's health conditions [14]
	• The terms *severely*, *morbid*, or *extreme* may be stigmatizing without adding precision to clinical documentation
	• Instead, describe weight in terms of BMI, such as *50-year-old man with class III obesity* or *BMI of 43* or *elevated body weight/BMI*
Suffering from/ afflicted with obesity/ underweight	• This terminology labels the experience of having a high or a low BMI as automatically negative
	• Many individuals with a high or a low BMI would dispute this characterization, and it does not add value to the documentation
Unable to visualize neck veins due to neck habitus	• The implication of this statement is that the patient's neck is large enough to obscure the contours of the jugular vein and that the clinician would have successfully located the veins were it not for the patient's neck habitus (and not, e.g., because the patient is volume depleted, making the neck veins absent in an upright position)
	• *Neck veins not visualized* is a simple alternative
Cachectic, thin, skinny, malnourished	• Person-first language is preferred instead of using the adjectives *cachectic* and *malnourished* (e.g., *person with cachexia/malnutrition*) when used in an assessment
	• These interpretive adjectives have no place in the physical exam, where a more objective description of muscle bulk may be indicated (*temporal wasting*, *atrophy of the large muscles of the extremities*, etc.) because cachexia is a clinical diagnosis combining the exam findings of muscle loss with or without fat mass loss and an underlying illness [15]; this terminology is best reserved for the assessment rather than the physical exam

5.1.5   Documentation of Obesity in the Problem List

Obesity is often added to the medical problem list (Chap. 8) in the electronic health record (Chap. 6), although prior research suggests that it may be less commonly added to the problem list compared to other chronic conditions [16]. Adding this condition to the problem list will significantly increase the visibility of this language in the patient's chart. Depending on the EHR of the patient's health system, the patient is likely to see these words then appear in their health summary on their patient electronic messaging portal and on every visit summary that they receive. Some EHRs allow the clinician to edit the text of problems that appear in the problem list while retaining ICD-10 or SNOMED CT codes associated with this problem. In this situation, replacing the text of problematic ICD-10 codes for obesity with a BMI description is a potential solution. However, regardless of this EHR functionality, clinicians should ask themselves what value adding obesity to the problem list is creating. While inclusion of obesity in the problem list has been associated with increased likelihood of discussion of obesity and referrals for treatment [17], there exists no high-quality data to suggest that the inclusion of obesity on problem lists results in improved health outcomes for patients with elevated BMI. Regardless of the clinician's decision to document obesity in the problem list, the inclusion of this language in either the clinical note or the problem list should not be a surprise to the patient.

A summary of key points to consider when documenting body habitus is shown in Table 5.3.

5.2   What Is "Normal"

5.2.1   Definition of Normal

A simple word such as "normal" can have a wide range of meanings in medicine. For this chapter we will be discussing the usages shown in Table 5.4 and not those pertaining to geometry (normal angles) or chemistry solutes (normal saline).

Normal, or taken further as a concept of normalcy or normality, does not have a single definition or even a consensus theoretical framework in medicine [20]. In

Table 5.3 Key points

• No surprises: if weight is discussed in the clinical documentation, it should have also been discussed in the visit
• If further classification of obesity is necessary for a note, use BMI, or the World Health Organization (WHO) classifications of obesity, rather than terms such as *severe* and *morbid*
• Patients strongly prefer terms such as *elevated body weight* or *elevated BMI* to *obesity*, *overweight*, or *fatness*

Table 5.4 Examples of dictionary definitions of normal and abnormal

	Normal	Abnormal
Oxford Dictionary [18]	Conforming to a standard; usual, typical, or expected	Different from what is usual or expected, especially in a way that worries somebody or is harmful or not wanted
Merriam-Webster [19]	1a: Conforming to a type, standard, or regular pattern: characterized by that which is considered usual, typical, or routine	Deviating from the normal or average
	1b: According with, constituting, or not deviating from a norm, rule, procedure, or principle	often: unusual in an unwelcome or problematic way
	2: Occurring naturally	
	3a: Approximating the statistical average or norm	
	3b: Generally free from physical or mental impairment or dysfunction: exhibiting or marked by healthy or sound functioning	
	3c: Not exhibiting defect or irregularity	
	3d: Within a range considered safe, healthy, or optimal	

healthcare, use of normal is often consistent with Oxford's and Merriam-Webster's first definitions as well as Merriam-Webster's definitions 3b, 3c, and 3d (Table 5.4).

5.2.2 Normal as Used When Discussing Laboratory Test Results

When discussing test results (Chap. 15), the patient and provider are likely both primarily interested in the "healthy" meaning of normal. For the patient, they typically want to know whether their test results have any impact on their health, such as prognosis, diagnosis, or treatment. In this case, a note may describe a test as "normal," meaning not signifying any health concern to the patient.

However, a laboratory test may also be referred to as normal or abnormal based on comparison to its reference interval (also called reference range). In some cases, these meanings (impact on health and comparison to a reference interval) are concordant, and in others, they are not. Accordingly, clinical laboratories generally describe a "reference range" or "reference interval" rather than a "normal range," as it should be the ordering clinician's role to interpret the test results as to their impact on the patient (Table 5.5). Reference intervals often represent a percentage (e.g., 95%) of a reference population (which itself may be not representative, depending on the original methods used).

Table 5.5 Normal as used to describe test results

Test results	Example	Documentation	Comment
Thyroid-stimulating hormone (TSH) 3.0 IU/mL Test: within the reference range Patient: healthy	A patient is evaluated for fatigue. The clinician orders a TSH. The results come back the next day, and the clinician adds their comment to the results online.	[Comment about test results delivered directly to patient online] Dear ____, Your TSH was normal. Sincerely, _____	Here the test as it relates to both the reference interval as well as the patient's health is considered normal. The writer does not make explicit what meaning of the word normal they are using, but it likely would be interpreted as healthy, and the patient can see that the result is within the reference interval.
White blood cell count $4.0 \times 10^3/\mu L$ Test: not within reference range Patient: healthy	A patient is evaluated for fatigue. The clinician orders a complete blood count (CBC), all of which is normal except for a WBC of 4.0, just below the reference range. The clinician sees that this patient has had several CBCs over many years, all of which have a similar WBC, and the patient has otherwise been healthy.	[Comment about test results delivered directly to patient online] Dear ____, Your CBC was normal. Sincerely, _____	Here the test result is not within the reference range, but the clinician is using "normal" in the meaning of healthy. This statement may be acceptable, but it may generate a follow-up question from the patient about why it is not within the reference range, which many patients will interpret as abnormal.
		Dear ____, Your CBC was within the reference range except for the white blood cell count. Although it is slightly low, I suspect this is your normal baseline and not a cause for concern. Sincerely, _____	This comment to a patient addresses both the reference interval and the assessment of whether the test result will impact the patient. This approach may take more clinician time; however, it may reduce time spent answering follow-up questions.
PSA 1.2 ng/mL Test: within the reference range of 0–4 ng/mL Patient: potentially has disease	Patient was treated for prostate cancer and had an undetectable PSA following treatment. Clinician orders a PSA for routine surveillance.	[Assessment & Plan] 1. PSA is now detectable, concerning for biochemical recurrence. I discussed with __, will place a referral to their medical oncologist for a consultation.	Here the reference interval and implication for the patient's health are discordant—the test being within the usual reference range is actually a potential sign of disease recurrence.

For example, a patient may have a white blood cell count (WBC) of $4.0 \times 10^3/\mu L$ at baseline, which is below a laboratory's reference interval of $4.5–10 \times 10^3/\mu L$. The provider may assess that this value is the patient's baseline and that it does not have any implications on the patient's health. Conversely, a patient may have a laboratory value that is seemingly normal, yet be highly abnormal for that patient, as with a patient whose treated prostate cancer has risen from being undetectable to now being positive, yet remaining within the reference interval which is based on people without treated cancer. In other cases, a goal laboratory value may be different from a reference range, causing distress for a patient to continually see their values not within range, despite being at goal, as with a patient whose individualized A1c goal is higher than the reference range.

5.2.3 Normal as Used to Describe a Patient's Medical Conditions or Exam Findings

While the word normal can be confusing when describing laboratory testing, it is likely not as alarming as when it and its implied counterpart, abnormal, refer to a patient's individual characteristics.

For example, if a clinician hears a heart murmur on exam, they will appropriately document it in the Physical Exam (PE) section of the note. If the other examined areas are described as normal, then the heart murmur will stand out as, by contrast, abnormal. Whether the heart murmur has clinical significance, however, may be uncertain. Similarly, basilar lung crackles may be atelectatic and insignificant, or they may represent volume overload or pulmonary fibrosis.

As with laboratory studies above, quantitative exam measurements may have discrepancies between a reference range (therefore abnormal by that criteria) and a goal for an individual patient. For example, a blood pressure of 90/50 could be described as abnormal in that it is outside the reference range but could be at goal for a patient with heart failure.

Because of the multiple potential meanings of normal (and abnormal), rather than documenting *normal* or *abnormal* for exam findings, it is more clear to document positive and negative findings.

5.2.4 Normality and Conception of Disease

The concept of normality has social input beyond scientific fact. For example, some conditions may not be diseases at all.

Not having enough of the enzyme lactase to digest lactose may be considered a condition, or even an illness, and it has a corresponding ICD-10 code. However, approximately 60% of humans do not maintain lactase—therefore lactase *persistence* may be more appropriately considered not normal (as in not usual) rather than lactase *absence* [21]. Labeling a person as "lactase deficient" implies there is something wrong with them—or abnormal—when in fact they may be perfectly healthy. Lactose deficiency being considered a disease is influenced by both cultural norms (whether lactose-containing foods are considered normal foods) and the composition of the reference group (a sample with lactase persistence being more common).

Some conditions are genuinely less common, but not pathologic. For example, fewer people have a preference for either the use of the left hand or no preference between hands when writing. This quantitative observation is not disputed, even accounting for the era in which people who prefer using their left hand were forced to use their right hand. In the current era, few clinicians would consider left-handedness abnormal in terms of health, even if it is statistically less common.

As discussed above, an "abnormal" BMI for many people may be healthy. Being labeled abnormal may lead to changes in self-perception as well as cause stigma from external factors.

5.2.5   Other Normal-Like Words and Phrases

As with *normal* and *abnormal*, there are other phrases for which providing more specific data or findings provides more clarity. *Within normal limits* is sometimes written in the physical exam, but does not necessarily have a clear definition of what those normal limits are. *Unremarkable* is sometimes used to describe family history or a physical exam, but also lacks specificity.

5.2.6   Summary

A seemingly simple, everyday word such as "normal" may be anything but simple when used in clinical medicine. There is no consensus of what normal means in the context of medicine, and there are several different common usages. When considering best practices in patient-centered language in medical notes, the word *normal* may still be used, but it is worth considering in what context the word is being used and whether there may be a better way to convey the intended meaning. Being more clear may in some cases lead the writer to eliminate the word entirely (including its counterpart, "abnormal") or to use the word with appropriate clarification as to its intent. Some of these concepts are similar to those discussed elsewhere in this book when using language that reflects behavior or choices rather than disease states or conditions that represent the wide variety of humanity rather than being contributory toward disease.

5.3 Conclusion

Using the guidelines discussed in this chapter, medical descriptions of body habitus in medical notes can be less stigmatizing, more patient-centered, and more accurate. Changing notes may not by itself change internal biases but may be part of a greater culture change in how healthcare professionals and society think about and discuss body habitus. Related to body habitus is the concept of how what is labeled "normal" is established and what "normal" means in different contexts. By being reflective about intent when using the word *normal*, healthcare professionals can use language that more accurately describes their meaning.

References

1. Flegal KM, Graubard BI, Williamson DF, Gail MH. Cause-specific excess deaths associated with underweight, overweight, and obesity. JAMA. 2007;298(17):2028–37.
2. Jayedi A, Soltani S, Zargar MS, Khan TA, Shab-Bidar S. Central fatness and risk of all cause mortality: systematic review and dose-response meta-analysis of 72 prospective cohort studies. BMJ. 2020;370:m3324.
3. Chung F, Yegneswaran B, Liao P, et al. STOP questionnaire: a tool to screen patients for obstructive sleep apnea. Anesthesiology. 2008;108(5):812–21.
4. Kottner J, Everink I, van Haastregt J, Blume-Peytavi U, Schols J. Prevalence of intertrigo and associated factors: a secondary data analysis of four annual multicentre prevalence studies in The Netherlands. Int J Nurs Stud. 2020;104:103437.
5. Fearon K, Strasser F, Anker SD, et al. Definition and classification of cancer cachexia: an international consensus. Lancet Oncol. 2011;12(5):489–95.
6. Gomez MR. The clinical examination in myology. In: Engel AG, Franzini-Armstrong C, editors. Myology. New York: McGraw-Hill; 1994. p. 751.
7. Inker LA, Titan S. Measurement and estimation of GFR for use in clinical practice: core curriculum 2021. Am J Kidney Dis. 2021;78(5):736–49.
8. Sabin JA, Marini M, Nosek BA. Implicit and explicit anti-fat bias among a large sample of medical doctors by BMI, race/ethnicity and gender. PloS One. 2012;7(11):e48448.
9. Puhl RM, Brownell KD. Confronting and coping with weight stigma: an investigation of overweight and obese adults. Obesity (Silver Spring). 2006;14(10):1802–15.
10. Fernández L, Fossa A, Dong Z, et al. Words matter: what do patients find judgmental or offensive in outpatient notes? J Gen Intern Med. 2021;36(9):2571–8.
11. Hagan S. E66.01 and our culture of shame. N Engl J Med. 2021;385(25):2307–9.
12. Puhl RM. What words should we use to talk about weight? A systematic review of quantitative and qualitative studies examining preferences for weight-related terminology. Obes Rev. 2020;21(6):e13008.
13. Volger S, Vetter ML, Dougherty M, et al. Patients' preferred terms for describing their excess weight: discussing obesity in clinical practice. Obesity (Silver Spring). 2012;20(1):147–50.
14. Pearl RL, Walton K, Allison KC, Tronieri JS, Wadden TA. Preference for people-first language among patients seeking bariatric surgery. JAMA Surg. 2018;153(12):1160–2.
15. Evans WJ, Morley JE, Argilés J, et al. Cachexia: a new definition. Clin Nutr. 2008;27(6):793–9.
16. Baer HJ, Karson AS, Soukup JR, Williams DH, Bates DW. Documentation and diagnosis of overweight and obesity in electronic health records of adult primary care patients. JAMA Intern Med. 2013;173(17):1648.

17. Banerjee ES, Gambler A, Fogleman C. Adding obesity to the problem list increases the rate of providers addressing obesity. Fam Med. 2013;45(9):629–33.
18. Stevenson A, Lindberg CA, editors. New American Oxford Dictionary. Apple Mac Software. Accessed 30 Jan 2023.
19. Merriam-Webster Dictionary. https://www.merriam-webster.com/dictionary/normal, https://www.merriam-webster.com/dictionary/abnormal. Accessed 30 Jan 2023.
20. Catita M, Águas A, Morgado P. Normality in medicine: a critical review. Philos Ethics Humanit Med. 2020;15(1):3. https://doi.org/10.1186/s13010-020-00087-2.
21. Wiley AS, Cullin JM. Biological normalcy. Evol Med Public Health. 2019;2020(1):1. https://doi.org/10.1093/emph/eoz035.

Chapter 6
The Electronic Health Record

Angad P. Singh (iD)

6.1 Introduction

Electronic health records (EHRs) are nearly ubiquitous and have fundamentally changed how medical documentation occurs, how it is used, and who can easily access it.

EHRs of widely varying types have existed for decades worldwide, with more rapid proliferation in the twenty-first century. They are standard in Australia, New Zealand, and large portions of Europe with Asia, Africa, and the Middle East having more varied implementation rates [1]. In the United States, EHR utilization skyrocketed after the passage of the HITECH Act in 2009, designed to promote the adoption and meaningful use of health information technology [2]. The associated financial incentives for transitioning to a certified EHR resulted in 96% of US hospitals and 78% of office-based physicians adopting an EHR by 2015 [3, 4]. This broad implementation meant that notes became more accessible (no more paper chart to chase down) and shareable with other members of the healthcare team in real time, offering a new set of opportunities and challenges alike.

Today's outpatient notes generally follow the SOAP format (Subjective, Objective, Assessment, & Plan). Although now a well-established practice, the SOAP concept only became popularized starting in the 1950s by Dr. Lawrence Weed, a pioneering physician who created the problem-oriented medical record [5, 6]. In Dr. Weed's approach, a patient's medical needs were best represented in the medical record by organizing them into a set of "problems," each of which had an associated Subjective, Objective, Assessment, and Plan section. Initially developed

A. P. Singh (✉)
Department of Family Medicine, University of Washington, Seattle, WA, USA

Department of Biomedical Informatics and Medical Education, University of Washington, Seattle, WA, USA
e-mail: apsingh@uw.edu

© The Author(s), under exclusive license to Springer Nature Switzerland AG 2023
C. J. Wong, S. L. Jackson (eds.), *The Patient-Centered Approach to Medical Note-Writing*, https://doi.org/10.1007/978-3-031-43633-8_6

to aid physicians in clearly reasoning through a patient's medical problems, its structure became the norm in medicine.

Although notes began primarily to communicate with oneself and other team members regarding medical care that was delivered, the ease of access from digitization quickly introduced additional audiences for clinician documentation, including coders, payors, quality specialists, researchers, and, most importantly, patients themselves (Chap. 2). As technology matured, it also became increasingly easier to share notes across health systems via interoperability and to communicate with patients directly using secure patient portals. The mechanisms for patient communication have continued to mature considerably, and interactions between patients and healthcare professionals will continue to evolve as we see higher use of real-time communication, such as text messaging or chat.

While there remains debate about who truly "owns" medical data, it is clear that patients have full rights to access their health record. This became further cemented in the United States with the passage and implementation of the 21st Century Cures Act that went into effect in 2021, delineating that no systematic delays can be put in place that prevent patients from immediately accessing key elements of their medical record, such as notes and lab results [7]. It was now clear: patients need to be able to access their health data as soon as information is available, sometimes seeing items like laboratory test results even before their care team.

In this chapter, we will focus on how the EHR can both facilitate and complicate the practice of patient-centered language. We will also discuss basic design principles to develop strong note templates based on the principles taught in the other chapters of this book.

6.2 Problem List

The Problem List, as first articulated by Dr. Weed [6], is the core thread tying together a patient's medical record. Problem lists coalesce the various medical concerns that affect a patient's care. They, however, come with their own challenges.

When considering the patient-centeredness of Problem Lists, we must first begin with the name itself. By classifying various factors affecting a patient's health as "problems," the problem list may inadvertently over-medicalize otherwise benign descriptors (e.g., transgender status) or render previous health issues (e.g., remote history of substance use) gratuitously persistent, creating opportunities for stigma irrespective of their current impact.

Therefore, it is important to share with a patient what a Problem List is and its purpose and that, despite its name, some conditions may not be "problems" in the common sense of the word. While there is no consensus as to what should be included in a problem list (see Chap. 8 for further discussion), Problem Lists should generally include chronic conditions or key psychosocial factors and, to minimize clutter, should generally not include transient low-risk medical conditions, such as a common cold. Note that there is no consensus about which psychosocial factors merit enough importance to include in the Problem List, but we generally recommend including only those that are directly affecting the care being delivered.

When considering diagnoses to add to the Problem List, it is important to articulate clarity without sacrificing patient-centered language. Examples for this are mental health diagnoses (Chap. 11), especially if patients are not in agreement with the assessment, or descriptors of obesity, which can carry social stigma (Chap. 5). It is important to ensure, though, that one remains accurate and honest in the Problem List, and one should not avoid necessary medical terms to the detriment of good medical care and communication. Honest discussion with the patient about what is on the Problem List and why, including how any included conditions affect their health, can improve a patient's understanding of their health and decrease misunderstandings about terminology and labels (see Chap. 8).

6.2.1   Problem Lists in the EHR

Problem lists in the modern EHR era have diverged from a purely clinical framework. They are increasingly being used to support the needs of regulatory, financial, and clinical quality stakeholders. Accordingly, many EHRs have linked problem lists with discrete International Classification of Diseases (ICD) diagnosis codes such that the clinician can only select items with linked ICD-10 codes to add to the problem list. This comes with its share of benefits but also its share of challenges when it comes to patient-centered documentation.

As a benefit, linking problem lists with ICD codes allows for a shared language across EHRs, health systems, and even countries since ICD is an international classification system. When shared naming conventions are used, EHRs can more easily exchange problem list data, making it simpler for patients to receive care across multiple health systems. For providers, they can confidently select billable diagnoses when using a linked problem list entry since billing relies on use of ICD codes. In these ways, problem lists can be a major satisfier for patients and providers alike.

The challenge with how EHRs have implemented medical problem lists is that they overemphasize ICD codes and underemphasize clinical concepts. As an example, a patient with a history of diabetes mellitus with neurologic, renal, and cardiovascular complications may have three separate entries in the EHR problem list (one for each complication) even though a clinician might classify all of them under one single problem heading ("diabetes mellitus") defined by an overarching clinical concept. One of the risks is that the patient story can become diluted since summaries of patient care are stored across multiple diagnoses.

The impact of ICD-linked problem lists in EHRs can be reduced by selecting a primary diagnosis in the Problem List around which multiple entries can be organized. Additionally, many electronic health records offer the ability for users to update the label of a problem to include patient-centered language in some user- and patient-facing interfaces. Updating these with more patient-friendly language where appropriate offers more inclusive terminology without sacrificing medical specificity with associated ICD-10 diagnoses remaining intact on the backend. It is also important to offer the ability to turn off sharing of a particular problem so it does not display in a patient portal, a common feature in the modern EHR. For example, patients with a history of an eating disorder can be triggered if they see a recorded weight and may benefit from the details of a problem not being displayed within the patient portal.

6.2.2   Problem List Versus Past Medical History

There remains a persisting, unresolved debate about what the differences and best uses are for a Problem List (which can include active and resolved problems) as compared to a Past Medical History. In general, Problem Lists in electronic health records include problems (i.e., ICD-10 diagnoses) that describe medical concerns that are ongoing or otherwise impact a patient's care and require regular consideration, such as a prior history of malignancy.

Active problems represent medical problems being actively managed, whereas resolved problems were generally impactful but no longer affect current health decisions (e.g., prior history of femoral fracture). Often, resolved problems are time-limited. A Past Medical History can generally be considered similar to a Resolved Problem List (many clinicians resolve problems from a Problem List *and* add them to a Past Medical History at the same time) although it may include additional diagnoses with minimal to no current impact on health status, such as remote illnesses from childhood.

A more detailed examination of the Problem List and Past Medical History sections can be found in Chap. 8.

6.2.3   Problem List: Best EHR Practices

EHRs can facilitate patient-centered documentation in several ways:

- Include an explanation in the patient portal as to what a problem list is, as patients may not understand that not all problem list items are actually "problems" in the common sense of the word. Alternatively, consider renaming the problem list—unfortunately there is not a consensus term to use instead, and EHRs may not have this level of customization.
- Have a method to easily display current and resolved problems. In Dr. Weed's original paper, resolved and current problems are displayed in two columns in such a way that one can readily see both and still distinguish them as different. If resolved problems are not easily found in the EHR, they may be missed. Retaining all resolved problems as active, however, may result in excessively long problem lists (see Chap. 8).

```
┌─────────────────────────────────────────────────────────────┐
│                                                               │
│   Problem:        Gender Dysphoria (F64.9)                    │
│                                                               │
│   Display as:     Gender affirming care                       │
│                                                               │
│   Overview:                                                   │
│   Current treatment: estradiol, spironolactone                │
│                                                               │
└─────────────────────────────────────────────────────────────┘
```

Fig. 6.1 Example of EHR alternative problem list displays

- If unable to select a problem list entry that uses patient-centered language, use the "label" field of a problem to include patient-centered language when appropriate (Fig. 6.1). The label field allows a user to include an alternate wording of the coded problem and may be accessed via a clickable button in the EHR; it may have various names, such as "Display" or "Display as," depending on the particular EHR. Display labels can typically be written as free-text and will show as the default wording in the Problem List instead of the coded problem name for most patient-facing EHR interactions, including viewing in the EHR portal or importation into the clinical note under the Assessment and Plan section.
- Minimize outdated terms or stigmatizing terms by either not allowing them, having explanatory material accompany them, or making them not display as the default or top choices when searching.
- Healthcare systems with sufficient resources should have workgroups or committees that review coded diagnoses for stigmatizing or outdated terms. They should also collaborate with their EHR and clinical lexicon vendors to systematically improve diagnosis imports and displays.

- As an example, if the diagnosis of gender dysphoria (F64.9) must be used for insurance purposes and there is no alternative code currently available, the EHR's alternate label field (if available) may be used. Here it is called "Display as." It is a best practice to discuss this usage with the patient as well.

6.3   The Outpatient Note

Modern-day SOAP note templates are generally composed of the following key components:

- Reason for Visit/Chief Concern
- Identifying Statement/"one-liner"
- Subjective: History of Present Illness (HPI); may also include relevant Medical History, Surgical History, Family History, Social History, Review of Systems, and Problem List

- Objective: Vital Signs, Physical Exam, Laboratory Studies, Pathology, Imaging/ Other Study Results
- Assessment and Plan

The digitization of clinical notes has made it much simpler to pull data from other places in the health record. In some cases, data is added automatically into clinical notes, which can be problematic without close review. Templates may pull in outdated, inaccurate, or visually disorganized data that can obscure the information pertinent to the patient's current assessment and plan and make it harder for patients to understand documentation of their care. In extreme situations, this can create miscommunication, such as when outdated histories and plans from older notes are "copied forward" and when other clinicians or patients are unable to find key information buried in extensive templated data.

Since ineffective communication contributes to the top causes of sentinel events, clarity in note writing and key information is a priority for quality patient care [8]. To aid in visual clarity, some EHRs have created the ability to collapse certain sections of the note, such as the Subjective and Objective sections, to make it easier for readers to access the often-buried Assessment and Plan section. As an alternative, one can consider using the "APSO" note format: Assessment and Plan followed by Subjective and Objective. One large health system in Colorado implemented the APSO note format across inpatient and outpatient sites, with the Assessment and Plan easily visible at the top of the note, resulting in high rates of adoption (94% of outpatient notes and 94% of academic hospital inpatient notes reviewed) and high levels of satisfaction for writers and readers of the notes [9].

6.3.1   Reason for Visit (a.k.a. Chief Complaint/Chief Concern)

The term chief complaint has been around since early medical journal reports in the 1800s [10]. From the patient perspective, the term "complaint" sounds as if the patient is complaining [11]. Although some may use Chief Concern as an alternative, a shift to using the phrase Reason for Visit (or Hospitalization, Admission, etc.) is more straightforward.

The Reason for Visit may be noted by a staff member, the provider, or directly entered by the patient via an EHR interface [12]. It is often simply a phrase offering a very brief descriptor, such as *chest pain*. Although it is included as a discrete item in many outpatient note templates and can be pulled in as an automated data field in some EHRs, there is no requirement for this. To minimize note length, it can instead be included as part of the HPI.

6.3.1.1   Best practices for EHR Reason for Visit:

- Consider not using at all; instead use the opening identification statement in the HPI which typically includes the Reason for Visit.
- If used, use the phrase Reason for Visit rather than Chief Complaint or Chief Concern(s).

- If available, allow the patient to directly enter the reason for the visit in their own words through the patient portal.
- Avoid the use of stigmatizing language (see Chap. 7).

6.3.2   HPI and One-Liner

A typical first line or identification statement of the HPI may include the patient's name, age, gender, relevant medical conditions, and reason for being seen. It is left to the individual clinician's judgment as to which pertinent medical or social history to include; stigmatizing diagnoses such as substance use disorder and stigmatizing social conditions such as homelessness, especially if not immediately relevant to the reason for being seen, may trigger the implicit biases of a note reader and unduly influence the quality of subsequent care the patient receives. Poor word choice (e.g., *IV drug user*) may compound the harm from such labeling. Identities such as race, ethnicity, and sexual orientation are almost never appropriate to include in a one-liner since they offer limited clinical value in the one-liner and can be disproportionately used with minority patient populations or certain clinical conditions without a biological basis. Chapter 7 discusses these issues further.

The organization of electronic notes is typically codified in templates, with many components automatically retrieved from data already stored in the EHR. For example, it is common to see an identifying statement for an ID that reads *[First Name Last Name] is a __ year old Female who presents for ____.* This nearly automated statement improves efficiency but does not necessarily improve clarity or inclusivity. Firstly, most modern-day EHRs allow easy collection of a patient's preferred or chosen name. With patients now being a key consumer of notes, it is important to input the name a patient uses ("What may I call you?") and include that in the note. It is also increasingly common to ask patients their pronouns and their gender identity rather than simply adding their listed sex from the record.

6.3.2.1   Best EHR Practices for the One-Liner

- If using a templated one-liner, be sure that accurate gender data is collected and entered into the EHR. A provider may know the correct gender in conversation, but the patient-provider relationship can be damaged by misgendering in a templated note that pulls in incorrect EHR gender information.
- Do not include templated race or ethnicity in the one-liner.
- Do not include language preference or proficiency in the one-liner. (It may be included elsewhere if relevant.)
- Do include a patient's preferred or chosen name; providers should verify with the patient, as other staff members may have collected the patient's name data.

6.3.3 Subjective (HPI)

There are varying practices for the HPI, from long-form paragraphs to bulleted items, which likely vary by practitioner, care setting, EHR capability, availability of voice-to-text/transcription services, and local medical culture.

One of the great debates of the Subjective section is the inclusion of various History elements and a Review of Systems. While neither is a required component in the United States for ambulatory billing since 2021 and inpatient billing since 2023, it is important to include key and relevant diagnoses and symptoms as applicable to the visit since they may be important for clinical reasoning. Doing so also ensures that the patient is heard and knows that their other medical conditions are being considered.

Co-creation of patient histories using Patient-Entered Questionnaires in which patients answer key questions in their own words is becoming increasingly common as well [11, 13]. While it can be a helpful reference, be sure to review the patient's answers with them instead of taking them at face value, documenting key highlights from a patient's answers in the HPI rather than an en bloc copy of a patient's responses. There are some exceptions, however, especially in the case of asynchronous virtual visits (sometimes referred to as "digital E&M visits" in the United States) where the patient purely provides the history via written format without any face-to-face or real-time communication. In this case, it is perfectly acceptable to offer verbatim wording from the patient with appropriate attribution. Assigning patient questionnaires in advance of a visit can streamline both the visit and the documentation process.

The Subjective/HPI portion of the note is a frequent source of potentially stigmatizing or negative language (see Chap. 7). Common issues include the use of doubting language such as *claims* or *insists*; the word *denies* (especially if used when referring to stigmatizing conditions such as substance use); misgendering (see also Chap. 3); and over-attribution (using phrases such as *the patient states* excessively throughout a note). Additionally, while quoting the patient in the medical note allows for inclusion of the patient voice, it must be done mindfully and with enough context. For example, writing that a patient has "pain all over" can be perceived as doubting their symptoms even if the intention is to better articulate the severity of symptoms.

With regard to the EHR, ensuring patient-centered language in a note writer's free-text or dictated narrative is not something the EHR can easily facilitate; however, many clinicians use field-entry elements within the HPI—these can be created with patient-centeredness in mind. For example, auto-generated EHR block elements for the Review of Systems frequently are phrased as *Endorses* and *Denies* for positives and negatives. Additionally, while the use of font differences (italics, color, size, bold, etc.) can make text more visually obvious, it can also compound potentially stigmatizing diagnoses, e.g., Review of systems: Constitutional: **obesity**.

6.3.3.1   Best EHR Practices for the Subjective/HPI

- Include a narrative section written by the patient if the EHR patient portal allows.
- Quote carefully or not at all.
- Ensure accurate pronouns if pronouns are used in templating.
- Use *positive* or *negative* or *has* or *does not have* rather than *endorses* and *denies* for pertinent symptom review.
- Do not require a review of systems—allow importation of ROS data entry tools if a provider prefers to use them, but maintain patient-centered language.
- When documenting social or behavioral health history, use patient-centered terms (see Chaps. 9, 10, and 11). For example, do not include a field called *illicit drugs*.

6.3.4   Objective

The Objective section generally includes a patient's vital signs, a physical exam, and studies such as laboratory tests, pathology, and procedural and imaging results. Modern-day EHRs allow a user to bring in much of this data automatically. The Objective section is one of the highest risk areas for clutter and duplication of information. To facilitate patient-centered documentation, it is important to offer focused findings that are relevant to the patient's care to maximize clarity. Having a good understanding of billing requirements can also minimize extraneous information.

When writing the physical exam findings themselves, the EHR often drives the method of entry and display. Users may use a combination of free-text entry, dynamic point-and-click tools, and pick-lists that offer pre-set exam finding options to write the physical exam.

- With free-text entry, it is prudent to avoid using a complete physical exam template that has been pre-filled since this requires the provider to manually delete any elements of the physical exam that were not actually performed. This risks the inclusion of exam findings that are inaccurate and, in addition to being fraudulent, can undermine patient confidence in the entire note. Instead, it may be easier to create pre-templated components of physical exam documentation that are then added individually.
- Use of point-and-click tools offers an efficient means for documentation but may offer overly generalized language that a provider cannot control, so be sure to include specificity wherever possible for maximal clarity. For example, "Right Breast: Mass present" is clinically insufficient and would be better described by adding location, relative size, and firmness of the mass, so it is important that providers add specific comments describing these features.
- Structured note templates may also use pick-lists that give pre-set options for ease. Be sure to review each option carefully and select only what is pertinent

and relevant to the patient at the time of the evaluation, free-texting any additional findings.

EHR developers should ensure that discrete field choices include only objective and non-stigmatizing language as discussed in Chap. 12.

Use of rich text features in EHRs is particularly helpful in this section. Consider bolding key findings to articulate a notable finding. Creating clear body system headers with underlining can make it easier for patients and other clinicians to follow your exam documentation. Take special caution with the use of colored font, though, as certain colors may be difficult to read for those with color blindness [14] and can increase stigma when used to document potentially stigmatizing conditions.

Whenever possible, avoid potentially unclear verbiage like "normal" or "abnormal," which are relative terms that can change from patient to patient (see Chap. 5). Remember, the patient did not go to medical school so they may not know what a normal or abnormal finding is. Also, precision is important here. Jargon may be both acceptable and appropriate (e.g., a *positive McMurray's test*) so long as other medical providers will clearly understand. Furthermore, one must remain objective and write accordingly. For example, descriptions of a patient as *obese, disheveled,* or *malodorous* may not be pertinent to the evaluation and may be stigmatizing for the patient.

EHRs are only as good as the data within them. This is particularly salient when documenting physical exam findings for transgender patients where available EHR tools may be inadequate and discordant with anatomy. Whenever technically possible, completing an organ inventory can help tailor EHR tools to offer more appropriate physical exam tools; inputting a gender identity can allow for EHRs to present all physical exam options, not just those restricted by male or female sex.

Beyond physical exam documentation, EHRs have simplified and, in some cases automated, the ability to include any number of lab, imaging, or other study results into the note. As highlighted previously in this chapter, the inclusion of large chunks of lengthy results can obscure more salient information in the note, so information should be added thoughtfully.

It can be helpful to consider which results need to be included in a note in the first place. As a good rule of thumb, only include test results that support the patient's care that day or support any associated clinical decision-making. Since results are typically saved elsewhere in the medical record, there is no specific requirement to copy detailed results into the note, and you may instead offer a brief summary of key findings (e.g., *Complete Blood Count: normal except Hemoglobin of 10*), including trends where helpful. This focused approach can offer insight into your clinical assessment for patients and care team members alike. (For a more detailed review on handling of test results, especially outside of a clinical encounter, see Chap. 15.)

Patient-centered language in the ROS and PE is discussed further in Chap. 12.

6.3.4.1 Best EHR Practices for the Objective Section of a Chart Note

- Be familiar with updated billing/coding guidelines—doing so will make it less likely to automatically have exam elements that are superficially commented on or lab results that provide no meaningful value.
- Exam documentation should not be pre-completed. Instead, findings should be freshly entered with an eye for inclusive language that is neutral and objective.
- Recognizing the limitations of free-text entry, point-and-click tools, and pick-lists for physical exam can help ensure exam documentation remains patient-centered.
- Templates with pick-lists should not include stigmatizing language (see Chap. 12).
- Use rich text/font differences with care, always being mindful of the potential for reinforcing stigmatizing language as well as accessibility considerations if introducing color.
- Include only pertinent lab and study result components given the high risk for adding significant clutter of limited value.

6.3.5 Assessment and Plan

In this section, audience is key. In the medical visit, one must communicate an assessment and plan to the patient, but also to other medical providers, and each audience has different needs.

The Assessment and Plan (A&P) is often delineated by individual problems or conditions. When adding diagnoses that may come with concerns from a patient perspective (e.g., obesity or terms related to substance use), share with the patient what medical diagnoses you are using for the visit so that mention of these technical words (which may or may not be appropriate) do not come as a surprise. Whenever possible, avoid stigmatizing disease terms and codes in the HPI, in verbal communication, and in the Assessment and Plan.

Many clinicians enter diagnosis codes for the visit and then import those diagnoses into the Assessment and Plan—while this practice is efficient, it may also bring in diagnostic codes that are out-of-date or stigmatizing. For example, a clinician can have a patient-centered, empathetic visit with a patient about the patient's substance use disorder, but that trust can be rapidly eroded if the patient reads "IV drug abuse F19.10 (ICD-10)" as the diagnosis in the Assessment and Plan, even if that term was not used verbally or in written patient instructions (see also Chaps. 10 and 13). Often these codes are linked to a medication and become automatically part of the encounter diagnoses (and therefore the Assessment and Plan diagnoses if imported).

Fig. 6.2 Potentially
stigmatizing diagnostic
codes can enter into the
Assessment and Plan
because of imported/linked
diagnoses

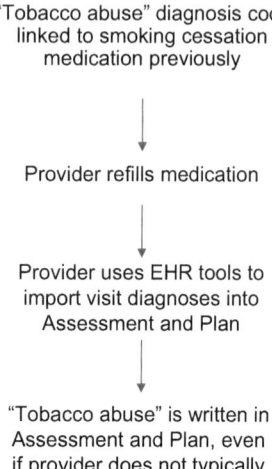

"Tobacco abuse" diagnosis code
linked to smoking cessation
medication previously

Provider refills medication

Provider uses EHR tools to
import visit diagnoses into
Assessment and Plan

"Tobacco abuse" is written in
Assessment and Plan, even
if provider does not typically
use that term and did not use
it when communicating with
the patient.

For example, when refilling a patient's medication for smoking cessation, if the prior diagnosis was "tobacco abuse," then that diagnosis will become part of the current visit diagnoses unless it is changed and also will become part of the Assessment and Plan if imported but not edited with free-text (Fig. 6.2). Providers may need to go back and change the current ICD code associated with the medication order or adjust the associated label, which unfortunately is an extra step and sometimes challenging to do if an order is already signed. In some cases, stigmatizing codes are unavoidable and it is always advisable to have a conversation with the patient (see Chap. 13).

In the name of efficiency, one can consider duplicating (or utilizing as a base) the patient instructions as the foundation of a note's A&P section, but this may require bolstering with additional medical decision-making discussion and adjustments to a more technical writing style for maximal clarity with colleagues.

6.3.5.1 Best EHR Practices for the Assessment and Plan

- If importing visit diagnoses or other diagnoses associated with medications or orders, ensure that the terminology is patient-centered. Change associated codes or update labels if necessary and able.
- If potentially stigmatizing codes must be used, discuss the rationale with the patient.

6.3.6   Patient Instructions

The EHR's patient instructions section should be written in plain, simple language (commensurate with the patient's literacy and numeracy) to describe what diagnosis has been offered and what the recommended options and next steps are.

While non-stigmatizing medical jargon is appropriate within a medical note, patient instructions should be written in a patient-centered manner using terms that match a patient's health literacy to ensure understanding.

6.4   Billing and Note Bloat

Problem Lists have departed from Dr. Weed's initial conception of problems as medical concepts. Generally now linked with ICD-10 billing codes, Problem Lists are repositories of diagnoses that describe a patient's care but also simplify classification of a patient's burden of illness and offer easier reference for commonly used billing codes for a patient's care.

While problem lists provide clinical value, there is no requirement that a problem list must be included in a note at all. Especially over time, problem lists can become bulky and contribute to note bloat when they are otherwise easy to reference in other sections of the EHR. Although problem lists can be helpful to organize a patient's care, consider leaving them out of the note altogether as they are often shared in their own section of an electronic health record's patient portal and on the patient's after visit summary.

Similarly, note templates may include templated Review of Systems and Physical Exam data that formerly were built in to support higher levels of coding, theoretically indicating more physician work and clinical complexity. However, these data can be pulled forward from prior visits, and documented findings may not reflect the exam done that day and thus misrepresent the care delivered while obscuring the key elements of the visit with sheer text volume. With the 2021 changes to ambulatory Evaluation and Management coding rules that now allow physicians to bill by medical complexity and time, it is prudent to forego the bulky Review of Systems and Physical Exam sections and document only what is clinically relevant in a more focused approach [15].

6.5   Notecrafting

The art of notecrafting and creating high-quality note templates in electronic health records is an undervalued but highly useful skill. Writing easy-to-read, aesthetically pleasing, and well-organized notes dramatically improves readability and makes it easier for patients and others to follow along.

Whenever possible, use a minimum note template to organize note content. A standard look-and-feel makes it easier for patients to follow key sections of the note from visit to visit and, as a side benefit, makes it easier for other note audiences to identify key information. Aesthetics represent a key and underappreciated foundation of note templates. Ensure the font type and size are easy to read and use colors carefully, paying particular attention to accessibility guidelines as noted above.

Consider adding a short, standard header at the top of all notes to convey key identifying information, especially patient-centered information such as a patient's preferred/chosen name, pronouns, and other key demographic information. Clearly delineate sections of the note with headers that are easily identifiable and reused from note to note. Resist the temptation to automatically add large volumes of text found elsewhere in the health record, such as medical histories, the problem list, or test results.

When writing the note itself, use EHR features like autocorrect to improve readability without adding keystrokes (e.g., autocorrecting "amox" to "amoxicillin," "BID" to "two times per day"). This also helps avoid error-prone abbreviations that have been shown to contribute to medical errors [16].

6.5.1 Best EHR Practices for Notecrafting

- Use a minimum note template to offer consistency in note appearance for patients. Aesthetics matter—develop the note structure to be pleasing to the eye.
- Create a short, standard header that conveys key patient information including preferred/chosen name and pronouns.
- Use autocorrect features in the EHR to reduce abbreviations, improve readability, and save keystrokes.
- Avoid the auto-inclusion of information easily found elsewhere in the chart in order to limit clutter and note bloat.

6.6 Conclusion and Future Directions

Patient-centered notes are the norm moving forward, especially in an era where patients have great transparency with respect to their medical chart. As discussed in this chapter, the EHR, when used appropriately, can enhance the patient-centered language principles discussed in other chapters in this book and allow for patients to be better represented in the chart. Care should be taken when EHR templates are built in order not to systematize stigmatizing language, and clinicians should be on the alert in case their EHRs have such language so that their notes do not inadvertently include it.

While it is always recommended to include the patient voice when writing notes, future directions include further steps in this direction. The OurNotes initiative from the Open Notes collaborative is a prelude to the future of patient-centered notes, where patients are actively invited to engage in the note writing process [12].

Systems are only as good as the design upon which they are built. Increasingly, artificial intelligence will be used to triage patient queries and co-create a clinician's documentation. However, we must remain attuned to what is written to ensure it is carefully vetted for clinical accuracy and patient-centered word choices. The same concepts apply to the use of scribes (both in-person and virtual) and dictation tools—scribes must be trained in patient-centered language, and their work must be verified, and dictation tools must not be built in such a way that stigmatizing language preferentially enters into the text.

Undoubtedly, new pressures and needs will continue to arise that will affect a clinician's documentation in the EHR. As each new goal or technology is introduced, EHR designers will need to remain cognizant of the need to maintain patient-centered language in order to provide the best possible experience for our patients and anyone who uses the EHR.

References

1. The Commonwealth Fund. What is the status of electronic health records? 5 June 2020. https://www.commonwealthfund.org/international-health-policy-center/system-features/what-status-electronic-health-records. Accessed 15 May 2023.
2. HHS.gov. HITECH act enforcement interim final rule. https://www.hhs.gov/hipaa/for-professionals/special-topics/hitech-act-enforcement-interim-final-rule/index.html. Accessed 29 Mar 2023.
3. Adler-Milstein J, Jha AK. HITECH act drove large gains in hospital electronic health record adoption. Health Aff (Millwood). 2017;36(8):1416–22. https://doi.org/10.1377/hlthaff.2016.1651.
4. Office of the National Coordinator for Health Information Technology. National trends in hospital and physician adoption of electronic health records. Health IT Quick-Stat #61. https://www.healthit.gov/data/quickstats/national-trends-hospital-and-physician-adoption-electronic-health-records. Accessed 15 May 2023.
5. Jaroudi S, Payne JD. Remembering Lawrence Weed: a pioneer of the SOAP note. Acad Med. 2019;94(1):11. https://doi.org/10.1097/ACM.0000000000002483.
6. Weed LL. Medical records that guide and teach. N Engl J Med. 1968;278(11):593–600. https://doi.org/10.1056/NEJM196803142781105.
7. HealthIT.gov. Information blocking. https://www.healthit.gov/topic/information-blocking. Accessed 15 May 2023.
8. Joint Commission. Sentinel event statistics released for 2014. Published 2015. https://www.jointcommission.org/assets/1/23/jconline_April_29_15.pdf.
9. Sieja A, Pell J. Successful implementation of APSO notes across a major health system. Am J Accountable Care. 2017;5(1):29–34.
10. Gillum RF. From papyrus to the electronic tablet: a brief history of the clinical medical record with lessons for the digital age. Am J Med. 2013;126:853–7.
11. Sykes DB, Nichols DN. There is no denying it, our medical language needs an update. J Grad Med Educ. 2015;7(1):137–8. https://doi.org/10.4300/JGME-D-14-00332.1.
12. Shucard H, Muller E, Johnson J, Walker J, Elmore JG, Payne TH, Berman J, Jackson SL. Clinical use of an electronic pre-visit questionnaire soliciting patient visit goals and interim history: a

retrospective comparison between safety-net and non-safety-net clinics. Health Serv Res Manag Epidemiol. 2022;9:23333928221080336. https://doi.org/10.1177/23333928221080336.

13. Walker J, Leveille S, Kriegel G, Lin CT, Liu SK, Payne TH, Harcourt K, Dong Z, Fitzgerald P, Germak M, Markson L, Jackson SL, Shucard H, Elmore JG, Delbanco T. Patients contributing to visit notes: mixed methods evaluation of Our Notes. J Med Internet Res. 2021;23(11):e29951. https://doi.org/10.2196/29951.

14. U.S. General Services Administration. Is there enough contrast between text and its background color? https://accessibility.digital.gov/visual-design/color-and-contrast/. Accessed 15 May 2023.

15. American Association of Professional Coders (AAPC). 99202-99215: office/outpatient E/M coding in 2021. https://www.aapc.com/evaluation-management/em-codes-changes-2021.aspx. Accessed 30 Mar 2023.

16. Institute for Safe Medication Practices. List of error-prone abbreviations. https://www.ismp.org/recommendations/error-prone-abbreviations-list. Accessed 15 May 2023.

Part II
The Medical Note

Chapter 7
The Chief "Complaint" and History of Present Illness

Cody Gehring and Renata Thronson

7.1 The Chief "Complaint"

Traditionally, the *Chief Complaint* is included at the beginning of the medical record of a patient encounter. The chief complaint may include a symptom, condition, or statement that describes why the patient is presenting for care [1].

7.1.1 The Term "Chief Complaint"

Although the word *complaint* has a medical definition—an illness or medical condition—the general public is more likely to understand the word *complaint* by its more common usage: an expression of, or reason for, dissatisfaction [2]. A patient reading a medical note may therefore interpret this term as the note writer believing that the patient is *complaining*. Some writers use the phrases *Chief Concern* [3] or simply *Concerns:* ___, which are less likely to be misinterpreted, although *concern* may be more likely equated with anxiety or worry rather than subject matter.

C. Gehring · R. Thronson (✉)
Division of General Internal Medicine, Department of Medicine, University of Washington, Seattle, WA, USA
e-mail: gehric@uw.edu; lrenata@uw.edu

© The Author(s), under exclusive license to Springer Nature Switzerland AG 2023
C. J. Wong, S. L. Jackson (eds.), *The Patient-Centered Approach to Medical Note-Writing*, https://doi.org/10.1007/978-3-031-43633-8_7

7.1.2   Utility

A counterargument in favor of keeping the phrase *Chief Complaint* is that it is simply medical jargon. Indeed, medical jargon is acceptable and often necessary in medical documentation—patients being able to read their notes is not intended to make clinicians replace all medical terms with lay language. However, even if accepted as medical jargon, the term *Chief Complaint* does not necessarily match its intended purpose: to describe the reason for being seen in a healthcare setting, which may be neither a complaint nor have a priority. For example, patients seen in the ambulatory care setting commonly have several items to address, without a single, "chief" agenda item. Furthermore, even if one uses the medical definition of complaint (an illness or medical condition), up to a quarter of outpatient visits are for preventive services such as well-child checkups [4]; calling such preventive visits a "complaint" becomes nonsensical.

Having a section of the note for the "Chief Complaint" may not be necessary at all. Its historical inertia is likely in large part driven by billing requirements under the Evaluation and Management (E/M) system in which the Chief Complaint (called specifically as such) was a required "element" of the medical history (the others being the History of Present Illness, the Review of Systems, and the Past Family and/or Social History). These elements were used in a complex formula to assign a billing level linked to reimbursement for providing clinical services, prompting coders to look for the Chief Complaint—which was required for all billing levels—as a separate line item. Claims could be rejected if the Chief Complaint was absent or deemed not specific enough (e.g., writing *Chief Complaint: Follow up* rather than including a symptoms or diagnosis).

However, in 2021, the American Medical Association (AMA) and the Centers for Medicare and Medicaid Services (CMS) in the United States eliminated the requirement for these complex formulas. The AMA Current Procedural Terminology® guidelines no longer mandate a "Chief Complaint" at all, instead requiring only a "medically appropriate history and/or physical examination" [5]. The CMS notes that the "Chief Complaint" may now be included within the History of Present Illness and is not obligated to be a separate section of the note [6]. Electronic health records (EHRs), healthcare systems, and medical education may take time to adapt to these lessened requirements.

If a separate part of the note (either within the note or as a separate EHR section) describing the reason for the patient's outpatient visit or hospitalization is nevertheless still deemed desirable (e.g., for quality improvement or other tracking purposes), then the phrase "Reason for Visit" or "Reason for Hospitalization" would be at once more encompassing as well as more useful.

Table 7.1 Examples of reasons for visit that may contain biased language

Reason for visit	Comment
Multiple complaints	This phrase may imply that the patient is difficult or that the multiple complaints are burdensome
"They told me I had to come in"	Quotations may be neutral but often express either doubt or an unspoken opinion about the patient. Here it may imply that the patient is not responsible

7.1.3   Chief Complaint (or Reason for Visit): Contents

If used, what is written in the Reason for Visit is subject to the same biases as discussed elsewhere in this book. Examples are shown in Table 7.1.

In some EHRs, patients may directly enter their own reasons for a visit. In this case, no more needs to be done other than confirm the accuracy of what the patient wrote.

7.2   The "One-Liner"

The introductory sentence or "one-liner" is often used to create a summary statement that primes the audience with the patient identifiers, past medical history, and reason for being seen—functioning like a news headline. However, as with a news headline, what it includes and omits may bias the reader. The one-liner may be a separate section before the History of Present Illness (HPI) or may be the first line of the HPI.

7.2.1   Inclusion of Medical Conditions

Certain medical conditions are often included in the opening statement of a patient note (Fig. 7.1). Whether to include medical conditions, and if so, which ones, is ultimately up to the note writer, and there is no consensus as to the best practices. For example, for a patient presenting with exertional chest pain, it would generally be considered helpful to know upfront their cardiovascular risk factors or whether they have a prior history of heart disease. How much detail to include for a medical condition depends on the context (e.g., for heart failure, the type, class, and possibly the ejection fraction may be important to document in the one-liner for a patient presenting to cardiology clinic, but they may not be needed upfront in the one-liner when the patient is seen at a different clinic).

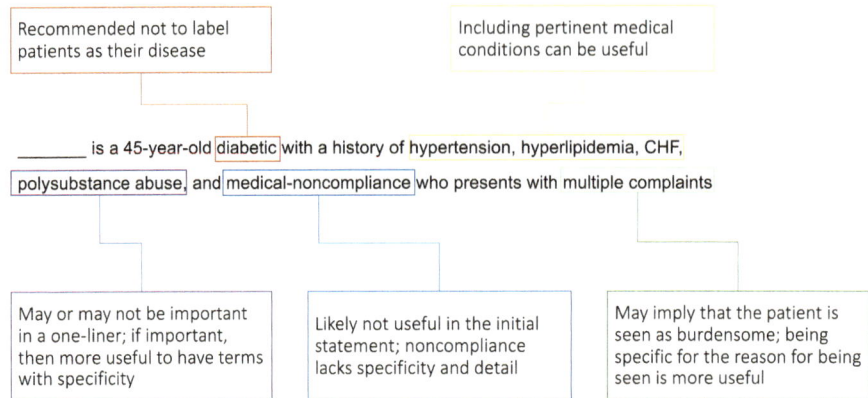

Fig. 7.1 The one-liner. Examples of potentially problematic language: medical conditions, non-compliance, and the reason for seeking care

Table 7.2 Examples of disease labels [7]

Disease label	Suggested alternative—examples
Diabetic	Person with diabetes
HIV patient	Person living with HIV [8]
Transplant patient	… patient with a history of liver transplant
IV drug user	… person with a history of substance use disorder…[a]
Sickler	Person with sickle cell disease
CF-er	Person with cystic fibrosis
Fibromyalgia patient	Person with fibromyalgia
Chronic pain patient	Person with chronic pain
Vasculopath	… history of coronary artery disease and stroke

[a]As with any medical condition, more detail may be included if appropriate to the clinical context; if the route of administration (e.g., IV) or the specific substance is critical to the presentation, then the note writer may elect to include these details in the one-liner; otherwise they may be discussed later in the HPI

If medical conditions are included, using the following patient-centered practices remains paramount.

Labeling: It is generally recommended to list medical conditions rather than labelling a patient as their medication condition (see Chap. 3). Examples are shown in Table 7.2.

Labeling is a complex phenomenon: A systematic review found that it can have both positive (e.g., community support, advocacy) and negative (e.g., negative behavior modification, social stigma) impacts, but that on an individual patient level, it more commonly had negative impacts [9]. Labels may vary in positive, negative, or neutral associations, which are influenced by individual and societal expectations. We generally discourage the use of "disease-first" terms such as *diabetic* or *HIV patient* and instead advocate for the use of person-first terms such as *patient with diabetes* or *person living with HIV*. In this way, a patient's medical conditions are not deemed inherent to their identity. This approach may reduce the risk of depersonalization, stigma, and other psychological impacts. For example, there is evidence that labelling a patient as their disease is associated with disparities in treatment: one study found that physicians who used the term *sickler* were less likely to adhere to national guidelines for pain management for patients with sickle cell disease [10]. Pertinent to the example in Fig. 7.1, the term *polysubstance abuse* may be stigmatizing, and such terms are associated with changes in care—for example, in one study physicians who read the term *substance abuser* as opposed to *having substance use disorder* were less likely to agree that the person needed treatment for their condition (see Chap. 10) [11].

Certain conditions such as substance use disorders may be disproportionately included in the one-liner, even if not relevant to a given clinical encounter. For example, patients with a history of substance use disorder, however distant, may still see this history featured prominently in their one-liner, risking erosion to the patient-provider relationship, as it may imply to the patient that the note writer views the patient's substance use as a core feature of the patient's identity. See Chap. 10 for further discussion of substance use documentation.

In some cases, patients may prefer to use terminology that is diagnosis-first: for example, a patient may identify as a deaf person or as a cancer survivor. Most importantly, we recommend eliciting preferred terms from patients and being open-minded to the likelihood of terminology evolving over time.

Medical noncompliance contains no information about why the patient is not taking their medications and may bias the reader to view the patient as uncooperative. Moreover, this may center the provider as the driver of medical care and the patient as a passive or unwilling recipient. It is better to address the patient's concordance with care recommendations in the HPI (see below) and Assessment and Plan (see Chap. 13).

7.2.2 Inclusion of "Chief Complaint" or Reason for Seeking Care

The reason for seeking care is commonly documented in the one-liner. The same principles apply as with the separately entered Reason for Visit. In Fig. 7.1, *multiple complaint*s may imply that the patient was burdensome or overwhelming—it would be more helpful to simply list the reason(s) for the clinical encounter.

A more patient-centered introductory statement could read as follows: ____ *is a 45-year-old patient with a history of congestive heart failure, hypertension, diabetes, hyperlipidemia, and substance use disorder who presents today for follow up of diabetes and chronic back pain*. The HPI could further discuss adherence barriers and details of their substance use disorder, if relevant. Alternately, one could simply write, ____ *is a 45-year-old patient here for scheduled follow up. Today we discussed the following...*, and then address the conditions in the HPI.

7.2.3 Inclusion of Personality or Other Traits

In Fig. 7.2, there are multiple issues that may contribute to bias and negative impressions of subsequent readers—both the patient and other healthcare professionals. At the outset, the writer labels the patient as *unfortunate*, which connotes a pitying view of the patient, who, in reading the note, may wonder what is so unfortunate about them. While empathy is important, there are other ways to convey this impression rather than labelling the patient in the first line. Even positively described traits (e.g., *pleasant* or *delightful*) should be either avoided or used with caution. While such terms may seem benign, it risks bias as to which patients a note writer decides to assign these positive terms. Additionally, the *delightful* patient may feel that they have been unnecessarily judged based on their personality [12] or that they have to live up to that standard at future visits, even if they are not feeling well or struggling in other ways. Finally, personality traits and terms to describe them lack objective definitions (the exception being specific psychiatric terms) and are unlikely to be relevant in professional medical documentation, especially in the first line of a note. There are opportunities elsewhere in a note (e.g., Social History, History of Present Illness, and Assessment and Plan) to describe a patient's resilience, struggles, barriers, values, and reactions in a way that offers details that are more specific to an individual patient's story and therefore more likely to be useful (see also Chap. 12 re: patient descriptors in the physical examination).

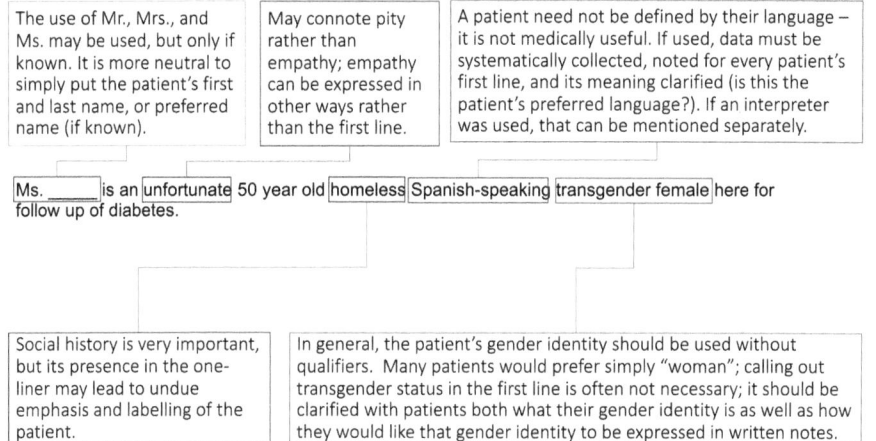

Fig. 7.2 The one-liner. Examples of potentially problematic language: gender, social history, personality traits, language preference, or proficiency

7.2.4 Inclusion of Social History

The Social History is an opportunity to document important aspects of the patient's life and circumstances surrounding their care, pertinent to social determinants of health as well as contributing to a holistic view of the patient as a unique and individual human being. However, despite its importance we suggest minimizing Social History in the opening statement, as it may be more likely to introduce bias than to provide useful clinical information.

In the example above (Fig. 7.2), housing status can be very pertinent to health—it may affect mental health, physical safety, the ability to maintain a regular sleep and diet pattern, access to a refrigerator for medications that require it, how a patient may be contacted in between appointments, and many other aspects of medical care. However, including housing status in the first line may bias readers. If included, it is better to not use housing status as a label (see above), but rather to describe it as a history item (e.g., ... *history of homelessness*), to avoid implying that the person is defined by their housing. There are many terms for housing, including *homeless, houseless/housed, unhoused/housed, undomiciled* versus *domiciled, having unstable housing* or *unstably housed*, and others. There is not currently a single consensus as to this terminology, and as with other terms, a discussion with the patient can be helpful (see also Chap. 9).

Other aspects of social history sometimes appear in one-liners but should generally be avoided. Inclusion of legal or incarceration status (e.g., ... *presenting from jail with...* or *prisoner* or *incarcerated patient*) may not only contribute to bias but also can impact trust between patients and providers. It is best to avoid including incarceration status in the one-liner. Lastly, unless it directly relates to the reason for the visit, the risk of bias likely outweighs the benefit of including occupation, sexual practices, immigration status, or marriage status in the opening statements of the note (see Chap. 9 for further discussion of Social History documentation).

7.2.5 Inclusion of Language Proficiency and Use of Interpreters

A patient's language(s) may be an important part of their social history. However, it is not beneficial in an opening one-liner. A problem with short-hand terms such as *English-speaking* or *Spanish-speaking* (Fig. 7.2) is that they are not specific or well defined. The reader does not know if the phrase ____-*speaking* means that the patient only speaks that language or speaks other languages but prefers that language. Further, ____-*speaking* does not describe the level of proficiency of any language. Only listing languages other than English may promote "othering" the patient outside a putative norm. In addition, a single phrase such as ____-*speaking* may also be overly reductive, as people often speak multiple languages with varying proficiencies.

If a preferred language is systematically collected, then it may be reasonable to systematically include that information in medical notes. The use of an interpreter is necessary to document. However, if preferred language and interpretation is documented, it is better to include it elsewhere in the note and to do so systematically (i.e., not only for languages other than English), for example, *Language preference: English. Interpreter used: No* or *Language preference: Russian. Interpreter used: Yes.* Locating this information at the bottom of the note may minimize bias.

7.2.6   *Inclusion of Gender and Sexual Orientation*

There is considerable bias related to gender, particularly experienced by those who are transgender or gender nonbinary. Transgender people and gender minorities experience significant health disparities. In one survey, 28% of transgender patients had postponed medical care due to discrimination, and 25% reported being harassed or disrespected in a healthcare setting [13]. Failure to accurately document gender identity furthers these disparities.

Note that it is often not necessary to document sex assigned at birth, transgender status, or other components of gender in the opening statement of a visit. In one study, patients reported a preference for gender and sex assigned at birth to be left out of one-sentence summaries [14]. For example, gender identity may not be pertinent to a visit for acute knee pain. However, if one does include gender in the one-liner, we recommend that there is a consistent approach across patients to avoid centering and normalizing gender majorities—that is, providers should also include documentation of gender when patients identify with a binary gender assigned at birth.

There is risk of including the wrong name, pronouns, or gender markers—thus, it is imperative that the provider takes care when using auto-populating texts in their documentation. Many EHRs have standardized sections in which sex and gender may be entered into the demographics section during a visit or asynchronously. Insofar as providers are able to influence the build of their practice's EHR, they should advocate for inclusive, unbiased terms in drop-down menus. Gender identification is also an excellent opportunity for shared documentation with patients (e.g., patient-entered information). Table 7.3 lists basic gender definitions to be aware of (see Chap. 4 for further discussion of gender and Chap. 6 for discussion of EHRs).

Not all patients identify within the gender binary (i.e., woman/man). For example, a patient may use different identifiers including they/them, transmasculine/transfeminine, or genderqueer. The best practice is to ask patients which terms they use and invite them to share in the process of medical documentation.

In the example above, the patient may identify as a *transgender female*, but it is also possible that they identify as simply *woman* and that for a given visit whether

Table 7.3 Examples of gender terminology [15]

Terminology	Definition	Examples
Gender identity	A person's internal sense of gender	Female/woman/girl
		Male/man/boy
		Nonbinary, gender-fluid, gender non-conforming, genderqueer, other
Sex	Historically referred to sex assigned at birth, based on external genitalia, chromosomes, and gonads	Male, female, intersex, other
Gender expression	Individual expression or display of gender. May be different than gender identity	Feminine, masculine, other
Sexual orientation	Sexual attraction; distinct from gender identity	Lesbian, gay, bisexual, pansexual, heterosexual, asexual, other

Note that these examples are not a comprehensive list, and terminology continues to evolve. It is most important to elicit preferred terminology from patients

or not they are transgender is either not relevant or even if relevant may not need to be called out in a one-liner.

Titles such as Mr., Mrs., and Ms. should also be clarified with a patient before use. For templated EHR notes, it is often more useful to simply write the patient's name unless the title is clearly known and systematically obtained.

Sexual orientation should generally not be included in a one-liner. Sexual orientation is better addressed as pertinent in the Social History; sexual practices should not be equated with sexual orientation and should be addressed depending on the clinical encounter.

The example shown in Fig. 7.2 could be more neutrally written as: ___ *is a 50 year old woman here for follow up of diabetes.* Other pertinent history may be explored further in the HPI or other sections of the chart or note.

7.2.7 Inclusion of Age Descriptors

Age bias is well documented in the literature. In one study, physicians were less likely to treat suicidal ideation in older patients compared to younger patients [16]. While age is typically an important clinical data point, we recommend against qualitative terms such as *middle-aged* or *elderly* (Fig. 7.3). Rather, we recommend writing the age quantitatively (years for adults, weeks/months for infants). Occasionally a patient's exact age may be unknown, or their documented age may be incorrect—those details may be noted as they may impact screening or other age cutoffs (example: *65-year-old (exact age uncertain) woman here for follow up of…*).

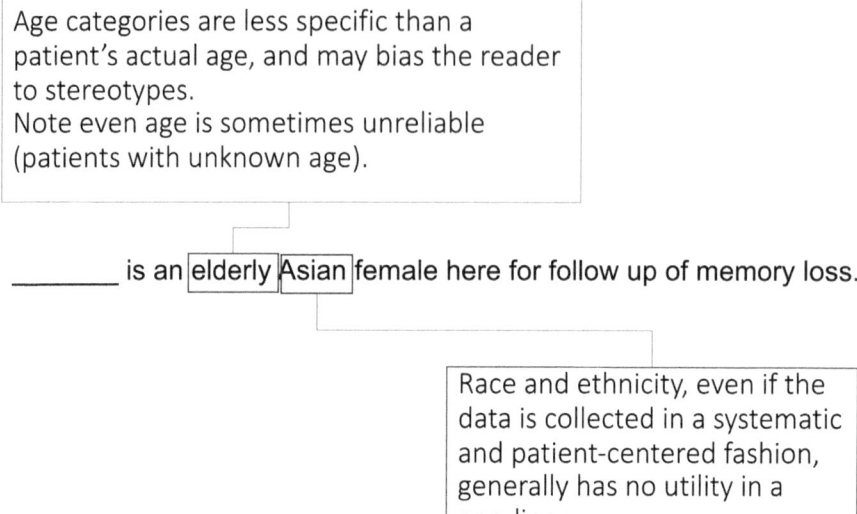

Age categories are less specific than a patient's actual age, and may bias the reader to stereotypes.
Note even age is sometimes unreliable (patients with unknown age).

_____ is an elderly Asian female here for follow up of memory loss.

Race and ethnicity, even if the data is collected in a systematic and patient-centered fashion, generally has no utility in a one-liner.

Fig. 7.3 The one-liner. Examples of potentially problematic language: age, race, and ethnicity

7.2.8 Inclusion of Race and Ethnicity

Historically, race has been understood as a broad category based on ancestral origin and physical characteristics, and ethnicity refers to a person's cultural identity (e.g., language, customs, religion) [3]. While there are ample associations between race or ethnicity and health outcomes, there is increasing awareness that race is a social construct and not a biological condition. There is no test or way to sort one person's race from another, and a person's self-identified race may be different from the racial assumption made of that person by others. Race and ethnicity have been further misused as a surrogate for ancestry [17]. Evidence suggests that there are more genetic variations within than between racial groups and that skin tone is not a surrogate for genetic predisposition to disease [18, 19].

Unfortunately, bias towards racial and ethnic minorities is pervasive throughout healthcare. For example, in one study, Hispanic patients with long-bone fractures were twice as likely as non-Hispanic White patients to receive no pain medications in an emergency department, even after controlling for other variables [20]. In another study, providers were two-and-a-half times likelier to use negative adjectives to describe Black patients compared to non-Black patients, even after adjusting for sociodemographic and health characteristics [21].

There may be very useful and helpful reasons to collect race and ethnicity data in healthcare. Such data can be used to address healthcare inequities. However, if collected, a patient's self-identification should be obtained in neutral fashion, with a wide range of possible choices (e.g., ethnicity should not be limited to *Hispanic* and *non-Hispanic* as is commonly done to adhere to the minimum United States Office of Management and Budget standards), including a write-in option, the ability to check multiple selections, and not synonymizing terms in order to force patients into multiple categories (e.g., *Black and African American* as a single category or *Latino/Latina/Latinx* as a single category). Such data, when accurately collected, may be stored in a demographic section of the chart.

In a medical note, race and ethnicity, as long as the history is taken in a sensitive manner, may provide helpful information and be written in narrative form in a patient's Social History section of the chart (see Chap. 9).

Race and ethnicity should never be included in the one-liner if not obtained in systematic fashion (e.g., if a provider makes an assumption about a patient's race or ethnicity based on their appearance and/or name rather than through systematic data collection via the EHR or at the time of patient registration). If race or ethnicity is documented in a one-liner, it should only be used in a systematic manner (i.e., do not include race only if non-White). On balance, however, the problems with data collection and the significant potential for bias far outweigh any potential clinical utility, so our strong recommendation is to not include race or ethnicity in the one-liner.

See Chap. 4 for further discussion of race and ethnicity in medical documentation in general.

7.2.9 The "Chief Complaint" and One-Liner: Summary

The one-liner can be very powerful as the opening statement to a medical note. As such, the healthcare professional writing a note must be very cognizant of this power and actively consider its potential for bias when composing the one-liner. These principles maintain importance whether the patient reads the note or not—it is not only the patients who may be affected by the impressions elicited from a medical note but also other healthcare professionals reading the note as well (see Chap. 3 for further discussion of the bias and affecting other providers). Table 7.4 lists key points for the "Chief Complaint" and the one-liner.

Table 7.4 Key points for "chief complaint" and one-liners

• "Chief complaints" as a separate part of the note may not be required
• Consider using the term "reason for visit" instead of "chief complaint"
• Recognize the risk of bias in one-liners
• Eliminate language or descriptors that are not directly pertinent to the reason for the visit
• Use person-first language
• Proactively discuss documentation with patients to ensure correct use of identifiers and terminology

7.3 The History of Present Illness (HPI)

The History of Present Illness (HPI) aims to describe the patient's experience of illness. The HPI is a foundation for clinical reasoning and diagnosis. While documenting a patient's narrative description of their illness experience may seem straightforward, it requires extensive training, in part because there are several different goals and processes required.

Presenting a Coherent Story A patient's history may be elicited in piecemeal fashion, out of chronological order, and with multiple symptoms and signs occurring at different times. The first goal of the HPI is to arrange the patient's narrative into a coherent story, typically in chronological order, that the next clinician can read and understand. For this reason, most histories are obtained by a clinician who then performs the HPI documentation. (There are evolving uses of history that is directly entered by the patient into the EHR or co-created with a clinician—see Chap. 6).

Combining with Other Data Sources In many situations, the note writer may appropriately bring in information from other data sources into the HPI. For example, a clinician seeing a patient in the clinic for hospital follow-up may include a summary of the hospitalization (information obtained from the medical record), including relevant tests and treatments, in addition to the patient's own narrative of what occurred related to the hospitalization and the history since discharge.

Editorial Choices The note writer makes decisions as to what other data to present in the HPI, which medical conditions to emphasize, and what other symptoms or signs are pertinent positives or negatives. This is a goal of the HPI (otherwise patients could solely enter their own history and fill out a survey of their review of systems) and has its own advantages and disadvantages. Medical history-taking and documentation in an HPI is at once a science and an art—it requires clinical judgment and is subject to the same clinical reasoning biases that are well described in the medical literature (anchoring, confirmation, premature closure, gender bias, among others).

Language Choices Every word that is written is a choice, whether thought-out or by force of habit. When documenting the HPI, providers run the risk of misconstruing or misrepresenting the patient's narrative in harmful ways. In this section we discuss how language choices in the HPI may be potentially detract from a patient's narrative.

7.3.1 Refusals and Noncompliance

A patient may decline a treatment recommendation or be unable to adhere to a treatment plan. The use of the words *refuse* and *noncompliant* are often used to capture this situation. However, these terms have two problematic issues. The first is

Table 7.5 Refusals and noncompliance: suggested alternative documentation strategies

Example	Example(s)	Alternative(s)
Refusal	The patient refused to take a statin	They did not take the statin due to concerns about muscle aches
Noncompliance	The patient never filled their prescription despite being reminded multiple times	They had a history of nausea from metformin and therefore did not fill the prescription
Noncompliance	The patient has been noncompliant with treatment and has multiple no-shows	She missed her appointments several times because she could not afford to miss work

language choice. Terms such as *refuses* or *noncompliant* imply a power dynamic in which the patient's role is to comply with the provider's wishes rather than participate in a collaborative or consultative relationship [3]. A more neutral way of describing the situation is to simply state what was recommended and that the patient did not complete that recommendation. Second, the reason for a patient's not doing what is recommended is critical to document. Patients may not follow through on a recommendation due to a myriad of factors. These include but are not limited to cost, mistrust in the medical provider (or system), side effects of treatment, cultural factors, competing priorities, and differences in health literacy. The medical chart provides an opportunity to highlight why a patient may or may not choose or be able to adhere to a treatment plan. By taking the extra step to find out and then document the reason a patient is unable to follow a treatment plan, the provider communicates unbiased insights into the patient's perspective and circumstances surrounding care (Table 7.5).

Nonadherence Versus Noncompliance *Nonadherence* tends to have less of a negative connotation than *noncompliance* [3], but connotations may change over time—it is possible that nonadherence will also develop more negative attributions. Both words can be avoided by more description of the situation and the patient's reasons for not "adhering" or "complying" with a given recommendation.

Defer Sometimes patients may defer a recommendation until a later date. If that is the case, it is helpful to state why, as well as when the recommendation is anticipated to be done (e.g., *The patient deferred the hernia exam today because their ride was waiting. They will do the exam at the next appointment.*). However, it is not recommended to use the word *defer* as a more polite version of declining altogether, as its meaning is different.

Decline Versus Refuse *Decline* tends to imply less power dynamic than *refuse*. As with nonadherence, it may still have a slightly negative connotation; to what degree may also evolve over time. One may also consider simply stating that the patient did not want to receive a treatment (e.g., *Patient did not wish to receive a flu shot today.*) or if there were a range of choices discussed, to document that (e.g., *Patient preferred to continue working on diet and exercise and not take a medication at this time.*).

7.3.2   Negative Language

Negative language can be introduced into the HPI both intentionally and unintentionally. Park et al. [22] studied 600 encounter notes and described multiple categories of negative language used by providers. These categories are discussed further in Chap. 3. In this chapter we highlight the negative language categories from this study that are commonly found in the HPI, as well as other examples.

7.3.2.1   Questioning a Patient's Credibility

A note writer can raise doubt about a patient's history, simply by the *way* in which the narrative is written, rather than directly addressing the issue. Park et al. identified this theme and found that word choice and selective use of quotations can imply that the note writer questions the credibility of a patient's history without directly saying so.

Words such as *supposedly*, *claim*, *insist*, or *apparently* are not required in an HPI. Rather, their insertion into the narrative is a decision made by the note writer, whether consciously or not.

Studies show that patients may react negatively to conventions such as "*patient claims*" or "*patient denies*," as well as any phrasing that dismisses the validity of the patient's perspective [12]. Within the HPI, there is generally a shared understanding that the source of the HPI is the patient unless stated otherwise. Therefore, it may not even be necessary to start each statement with *patient reports/states*, though this is a more neutral use of language.

Quotations are no longer purely a neutral recounting of verbatim speech. The decision to quote a patient directly is an active choice on the part of the note writer. Quotations can serve as a means of reflecting a patient's statements during a visit. However, in modern usage, quotations may be interpreted as expressing doubt or questioning a patient's history or interpretation of that history. In other circumstances, it may perpetuate negative stereotypes about a patient. Park et al. also demonstrated that the use of quotations for vernacular English may be used in a way that stereotypes or looks down on a patient's health literacy [22]. While quotations may sometimes have a role for conveying important context or capturing a patient's intent, often they are misinterpreted in a harmful way.

Quotes are not uniformly used as expressions of doubt, however—they are highly contextual. For example, palliative care discussions may use quotations in a patient-centered way, as one of the main goals is to elicit a patient or family member's values, hopes, fears, and goals. In those settings a direct quotation may capture that spirit better than paraphrasing. In other situations, a patient's description of their symptoms may be so apt that the clinician's narrative cannot do it justice, or it may support clinical reasoning (e.g., "worse headache of my life"). In psychiatry, direct quotations are often a useful way to show a patient's mental status. There may also be cases in which for medical-legal reasons direct quotations may be used, such as if a patient is threatening violence or there has been significantly disruptive behavior (see Chap. 14).

In general, however, because quotations often imply doubt, when considering quoting a patient directly, it is recommended to stop and assess whether the intention is to better capture the patient's narrative or express doubt—if the latter, then it should be avoided, and paraphrasing may be more appropriate.

In some cases, a clinician will write that a patient is a *poor historian*. The astute observer will note that the person taking the history is the historian and not the subject of the history [23, 24]. It is a better practice not to use this phrase.

Avoiding words that question credibility does not mean that a clinician should not question a patient's conclusions or interpretations. In fact, it is often the clinician's responsibility to do just that—patients seek healthcare for a professional consultation and care, not to confirm their own diagnostic impressions. Rather, it is more appropriate to address any conflicts between the patient's interpretation and the clinician in the Assessment and Plan (see also Chap. 13) and to do so in straightforward fashion.

Table 7.6 summarizes expressions of doubt and suggested alternative strategies.

7.3.2.2   Disapproval, Difficult Patients, and Minimizing Patient Autonomy

Park et al. describe three other themes of negative language: disapproval, difficult patient, and unilateral decisions. In all these situations, there is a conflict between the note writer and the patient with regard to what they believe is the right decision or conclusion for a clinical situation. These themes tend to involve some aspect of the interaction or decision-making, not just the history itself. Word choice may show disapproval of a patient's views, such as the use of *adamant* and *insist* (used in a different context than the credibility questioning above). Repetition words such as *still* and *again* may show frustration on the provider's part and cast judgment on a patient's choices or behaviors. A paternalistic decision-making style may supplant patient autonomy. Table 7.7 shows examples of these word choices and suggested alternative strategies. Some of this language may also occur in the Assessment and Plan (also discussed in Chap. 13). Other language suggests that a patient themselves is difficult rather than framing the situation as a difficult encounter or challenging conversation (for further discussion, see Chap. 14).

Table 7.6 Expressions of doubt or questioning a patient's credibility by language and use of quotations

HPI—questioning credibility	HPI—alternative	Assessment and plan—alternative	Comment
He insists that nicotine patches "don't work for him"[a]	He tried the nicotine patch several times, but it did not reduce his craving	n/a	This can be reported more neutrally without the word *insists* or the use of quotations
She says the flu shot "gave me the flu"	She felt that the flu shot gave her the flu. She had flu-like symptoms about 2 days after the flu shot last year	We discussed that although she felt that the flu vaccine gave her the flu, that I thought it was more likely that she either developed side effects from the vaccine, or coincidentally caught another viral infection	The patient's interpretation can be written neutrally, without quotations
			More details can provide insight into the patient's interpretation
			The Assessment and Plan can document the discussion between the provider and the patient as to the different conclusions as to the causal nature of the flu vaccine and the patient's symptoms
They claim that someone stole the medications	They reported their medications stolen from their locker last week		This can be written more neutrally without the word *claim*
He supposedly had a seizure but apparently never lost consciousness	He describes his seizure as having had full-body shaking for 1–2 min. He did not lose consciousness during the episode	Although some seizure phenotypes do not involve loss of consciousness, generalized tonic-clonic seizures typically do. I discussed that I recommended we also explore other causes of his symptoms	The words *supposedly* and *apparently* express doubt. Rather, the history can be documented neutrally, and the differences in interpretation between the patient and the clinician can be discussed in the A/P
Patient states that pain is "10/10"	Pain is 10/10		Use of quotations is not necessary

[a]Example is modified from Park et al. [22]

7.3.3   Denials, Endorsements, and Failures

Much of the negative language discussed above belies an underlying attitude or judgment on the note writer's part that comes out through the use of word choice or quotations. These word choices can not only potentially damage the patient-provider relationship when the patient reads such notes, but it can bias the next clinician reading the note.

Table 7.7 Disapproval, difficult patients, and minimizing patient autonomy

HPI—disapproving language	HPI—suggested alternative	Comment
This is the third time ___ presents for this complaint, despite my telling them that it is not cardiac	___ presents today for chest pain. We evaluated this at the last two appointments—I felt that it was noncardiac. Today the symptoms are…	If the fact that the concern is recurrent is important, it can be stated more neutrally
		The word *complaint* may be neutral to a clinician but more negative to a patient
		Despite implies a degree of disapproval
They are adamant that they have a candida infection	They believe that their symptoms are due to a candida infection because…	This patient belief can be stated more neutrally without the word *adamant*. Reasons for the patient's belief may be helpful to elicit and understand
He perseverates on the positive ANA test again at this visit	He requests an ANA test	The words *perseverates* and *again* are unnecessary. If the chronicity of the discussion is felt important to document, a summary of the discussion could be described in the A/P
She did not follow through with the referral even though I instructed her to do so many times	She has not scheduled an appt with ___ yet because …	The phrasing here implies a lack of shared decision-making—the clinician gives an instruction, and the patient is expected to follow through with it
		What the patient has or has not done can be stated neutrally. Reasons for the patient's choices can be explored and documented

However, some medical jargon can be more neutral to healthcare professionals but be interpreted in a negative fashion by patients who are not as familiar with these terms. These terms might not be associated with underlying biases but should still be considered carefully. In most cases, the terms, even if not used in a biased manner, may not be particularly useful in the first place—in other words, they are jargon that are not necessary because they do not have strict medical definitions nor add value in terms of disease description or classification.

Failure: Treatment failure is a common medical term, used in research and other settings to describe an unsuccessful treatment or other course of action. However, if used, it is better to make clear that the treatment is the failure, not the patient themselves. For many patients, participating in healthcare is a challenging experience. Some patients have had negative healthcare experiences and have also been unsuccessful in achieving their healthcare goals—*failure* has such a negative connotation that it can be discouraging to patients to be described as such.

Table 7.8 shows examples of language that is often not biased in origin but may have negative patient impacts.

An overall more neutral approach is shown in Table 7.9.

Table 7.8 Denials, endorsements, and failures—medical jargon that may not be biased but still have negative patient impacts

Example	Implication	Alternative(s)
Patient denies injection drug use.	The patient is being interrogated	Patient does not use injection drugs
Patient admits to missing medication doses	The patient reveals this information begrudgingly	Patient misses their __ dose on average of once a week
Patient endorses chest pain	Declaring approval of	Patient has chest pain
Patient failed treatment	It is the patient's fault that treatment was not successful	The medication failed to control the patient's symptoms
		The patient's condition did not respond to the treatment

Table 7.9 Example of HPI with and without the use of endorse, deny, and failure

HPI—using endorsements, denials, failures	HPI—without endorsements, denials, failures
__ presents today with upper abdominal pain	___ presents today with upper abdominal pain
They report 4 weeks of epigastric region pain, 6/10 at its worst. They report radiation up into the chest. Symptoms are worse after meals. They deny fever, nausea, vomiting, or shortness of breath. They endorse constipation and drinking alcohol. They *failed* attempted lifestyle changes including raising the head of the bed and avoiding spicy foods. They *admit* to taking NSAIDs for back problems. They *deny* drug use	____ gradually developed upper abdominal pain starting 4 weeks ago. It is 6/10 in severity at its worst, radiates superiorly into the chest, and is worse after meals. They have constipation, unchanged from baseline. They do not have nausea, vomiting, fever, weight loss, or shortness of breath. They raised the head of the bed and have been avoiding spicy foods, without resolution of symptoms
	They have been taking NSAIDs for chronic back problems
	Cigarette use: none. Alcohol: one glass of wine with dinner. Other substance use: none

7.3.4   Positive Language

We have so far discussed the potential harm posed by using negative language; however, the goal is not simply to replace negative language with positive language. Rather, unnecessary positive language and implied praise may also show bias and pose a risk to the patient-provider relationship. For example, in one study, a patient commented after reading their note: "It feels condescending, even when the comment is positive, when a doctor judges your personal character based on 5 minutes in an exam room. I feel like I'm reading my high school report card…assumptions being made, maybe based on race, gender, weight, etc." [12]. Examples of problematic positive language include complimenting the patient (____ *is a delightful*

62-year-old patient) (see discussion of one-liners above). In this case, the risk to an individual patient is that they may feel judged or compelled to please the provider in order to be deemed *delightful*. The risk on a systemic level is whether patients are given these positive labels in a biased fashion, as words such as *delightful* and *pleasant* lack specificity—what is delightful to one person may be different to another. Healthcare professionals in general should not be in the business of judging a person as pleasant or unpleasant.

There may be situations in which an aspect of a patient's character is enlightening or helpful to their care. Medical notes do not have to be completely devoid of a sense of the patient as a person. Rather than labelling a patient as *delightful*, or *courageous*, or *pleasant*, however, it would be more useful to describe what aspect of the patient's behavior or attitude is worth describing. For example, a provider may note a patient's resilience in working on exercise in the following example: __ *and I have been working together on their exercise goals for the past year. They have had setbacks with multiple injuries but I commended them today on their persistence and resilience—they have now found a new exercise routine that is more accommodating for their joint problems.*

7.3.5 Medical Conditions and Social History in the HPI

The HPI often includes information that may be otherwise located in other parts of the EHR or in separate sections of the note, including medical conditions (past or current medical history), habits, social history, and review of systems.

Language issues associated with these other history elements are reviewed in Chaps. 8, 9, 10, 11, and 12. Common issues include labelling patients as their diseases (similar to the one-liner discussion above), sexual history terms, and substance use terms. Inclusion of social history may be helpful but can also be unnecessarily harmful—one study found that vignettes that included language that implied socioeconomic status (e.g., *hanging out with friends outside McDonald's*) were associated with less aggressive pain management [25]. In most cases, including such stereotyped descriptions does not add to clinical reasoning.

Table 7.10 shows key points for patient-centered language in the HPI.

Table 7.10 Key points for patient-centered language in the HPI

• Recognize the impact of positive and negative language in documentation
• Use neutral terminology whenever possible
• Quotations may often have negative connotations and should be used with caution
• If you would not say it to your patient in person, it probably does not belong in the medical record

7.4 Summary

In this chapter, we highlighted circumstances in which bias and mistrust can be introduced into the "chief complaint," one-liner, and HPI. While it may feel challenging to maintain a patient-centered note, we suggest using this simple litmus test for documentation: anything that would not be said to a patient directly probably should not be in the medical note. Rather than conforming to a simple what-to-avoid list, now that patients are reading medical notes, it is an opportunity to reinforce authenticity, objectivity, trust, and collaboration between clinicians and patients. Language will continue to evolve over time, and partnering with patients will enable healthcare professionals to keep pace.

References

1. Peterson MC, Holbrook JH, Von Hales D, Smith NL, Staker LV. Contributions of the history, physical examination, and laboratory investigation in making medical diagnoses. West J Med. 1992;156(2):163–5.
2. Stevenson A, Lindberg CA, editors. New American Oxford Dictionary. Apple Mac Software. Accessed 6 Feb 2023.
3. Frey T, Young RK. Correct and preferred usage. In: AMA manual of style. Oxford: Oxford University Press; 2020. p. 505–50. https://doi.org/10.1093/JAMA/9780190246556.003.0011.
4. Centers for Disease Control and Prevention. National Center for Health Statistics. Characteristics of office-based physician visits. 2018. https://www.cdc.gov/nchs/products/databriefs/db408.htm#section_3. Accessed 6 Feb 2023.
5. CPT® Evaluation and Management. Office or other outpatient (99202-99215) and prolonged services (99354, 99355, 99355, 99417) code and guideline changes. https://www.ama-assn.org/system/files/2019-06/cpt-office-prolonged-svs-code-changes.pdf. Accessed 6 Feb 2023.
6. Centers for Medicare & Medicaid Services. Medicare learning network. MLN006764 January 2022. Evaluation and Management Services Guide. https://www.cms.gov/outreach-and-education/medicare-learning-network-mln/mlnproducts/downloads/eval-mgmt-serv-guide-icn006764.pdf. Accessed 6 Feb 2023.
7. Preferred Terms for Select Population Groups & Communities. Gateway to health communication. CDC. https://www.cdc.gov/healthcommunication/Preferred_Terms.html. Accessed 4 Dec 2022.
8. Centers for Disease Control. A guide to talking about HIV. https://www.cdc.gov/stophivtogether/library/stop-hiv-stigma/fact-sheets/cdc-lsht-stigma-factsheet-language-guide.pdf. Accessed 14 May 2023.
9. Sims R, Michaleff ZA, Glasziou P, Thomas R. Consequences of a diagnostic label: a systematic scoping review and thematic framework. Front Public Health. 2021;9:725877. https://doi.org/10.3389/fpubh.2021.725877.
10. Glassberg J, Tanabe P, Richardson L, Debaun M. Among emergency physicians, use of the term "Sickler" is associated with negative attitudes toward people with sickle cell disease. Am J Hematol. 2013;88(6):532–3.
11. Kelly JF, Westerhoff CM. Does it matter how we refer to individuals with substance-related conditions? A randomized study of two commonly used terms. Int J Drug Policy. 2010;21(3):202–7.

12. Fernández L, Fossa A, Dong Z, Delbanco T, Elmore J, Fitzgerald P, Harcourt K, Perez J, Walker J, DesRoches C. Words matter: what do patients find judgmental or offensive in outpatient notes? J Gen Intern Med. 2021;36(9):2571–8. https://doi.org/10.1007/s11606-020-06432-7.
13. Grant JM, Mottet LA, Tanis J, Harrison J, Herman JL, Keisling M. Injustice at every turn: a report of the National Transgender Discrimination Survey. Washington, DC: National Center for Transgender Equality and National Gay and Lesbian Task Force; 2011.
14. Alpert AB, Mehringer JE, Orta SJ, Redwood E, Hernandez T, Rivers L, Manzano C, Ruddick R, Adams S, Cerulli C, Operario D, Griggs JJ. Experiences of transgender people reviewing their electronic health records, a qualitative study. J Gen Intern Med. 2023;38(4):970–7. https://doi.org/10.1007/s11606-022-07671-6.
15. Terminology and definitions. Gender Affirming Health Program. https://transcare.ucsf.edu/guidelines/terminology. Accessed 22 Nov 2022.
16. Uncapher H, Areán PA. Physicians are less willing to treat suicidal ideation in older patients. J Am Geriatr Soc. 2000;48(2):188–92. https://doi.org/10.1111/j.1532-5415.2000.tb03910.x.
17. Lu C, Ahmed R, Lamri A, Anand SS. Use of race, ethnicity, and ancestry data in health research. PLoS Glob Public Health. 2022;2(9):e0001060. https://doi.org/10.1371/journal.pgph.0001060.
18. Amutah C, Greenidge K, Mante A, Munyikwa M, Surya SL, Higginbotham E, Jones DS, Lavizzo-Mourey R, Roberts D, Tsai J, Aysola J. Misrepresenting race—the role of medical schools in propagating physician bias. N Engl J Med. 2021;384(9):872–8. https://doi.org/10.1056/NEJMms2025768.
19. Witherspoon DJ, Wooding S, Rogers AR, Marchani EE, Watkins WS, Batzer MA, Jorde LB. Genetic similarities within and between human populations. Genetics. 2007;176(1):351–9. https://doi.org/10.1534/genetics.106.067355.
20. Todd KH, Samaroo N, Hoffman JR. Ethnicity as a risk factor for inadequate emergency department analgesia. JAMA. 1993;269(12):1537–9.
21. Sun M, Oliwa T, Peek ME, Tung EL. Negative patient descriptors: documenting racial bias in the electronic health record. Health Aff (Millwood). 2022;41(2):203–11. https://doi.org/10.1377/hlthaff.2021.01423.
22. Park J, Saha S, Chee B, Taylor J, Beach MC. Physician use of stigmatizing language in patient medical records. JAMA Netw Open. 2021;4(7):e2117052. https://doi.org/10.1001/jamanetworkopen.2021.17052.
23. Tiemstra J. The poor historian. Acad Med 2009;84(6):723. https://doi.org/10.1097/ACM.0b013e3181a43e28.
24. Lajeunesse M. Language that disempowers patients: the doctor is the poor historian. BMJ. 2022;377:o1296. https://doi.org/10.1136/bmj.o1296.
25. Goddu AP, O'Conor KJ, Lanzkron S, Saheed MO, Saha S, Peek ME, Haywood C Jr, Beach MC. Do words matter? Stigmatizing language and the transmission of bias in the medical record. J Gen Intern Med. 2018;33(5):685–91. Erratum in: J Gen Intern Med. 2019;34(1):164. https://doi.org/10.1007/s11606-017-4289-2.

Chapter 8
The Problem List and Past Medical History

Sarah Leyde and Margaret Isaac

8.1 Introduction

The primary function of the problem list is to distill the patient's health issues into a snapshot of need-to-know information, enabling the treating clinician to provide high-quality medical care. When done well, the problem list can improve not only clinician efficiency but also patient safety. Medical conditions included on the problem list are more likely to be addressed at future visits [1, 2]. For example, one study demonstrated that documentation of heart failure on the problem list is associated with an increased likelihood of prescription of goal-directed medical therapy [3]. Despite its benefits, the problem list lacks standardization and is frequently incomplete [4–7]. In recent years, general guidance has been suggested for creating and maintaining the problem list, but there is still no clear consensus regarding what diagnoses and other health issues should be included [8, 9].

The 21st Century Cures Act mandates that patients are offered access to their electronic health record (EHR) [10]. The literature suggests that the majority of patients view access to their medical records favorably and benefit from increased trust in their clinician, greater understanding of their care plans, and a feeling of greater control over their medical care [11–13]. However, some patients feel judged or offended by what they read because of errors, surprise information, labeling, or language suggestive of disrespect (Chap. 3) [14]. Concerningly, qualitative analyses of notes found that stigmatizing language is more common in notes written about Black patients and among patients with diabetes, substance use disorders, and chronic pain [15–17].

S. Leyde (✉) · M. Isaac
Division of General Internal Medicine, Department of Medicine, University of Washington, Seattle, WA, USA
e-mail: sleyde@uw.edu; misaac@uw.edu

© The Author(s), under exclusive license to Springer Nature Switzerland AG 2023
C. J. Wong, S. L. Jackson (eds.), *The Patient-Centered Approach to Medical Note-Writing*, https://doi.org/10.1007/978-3-031-43633-8_8

For clinicians tasked with curating the problem list, patient access to the electronic health record introduces both challenges and opportunities. How can we choose diagnostic codes that promote accuracy and also avoid stigma? What happens when the clinician and patient disagree on which problems belong on the problem list? How can we empower patients to contribute to their problem list to ensure accuracy? In this chapter, we will examine the implications of the patient-facing electronic health record on the problem list and discuss opportunities for clinicians and patients to work together to curate a meaningful, accurate problem list that benefits patient care. We focus on the problem list as a stand-alone element in the electronic health record (the use of problems within a note, as in the Assessment and Plan, is discussed in Chap. 13).

8.2 Origins of the Problem List

The problem list was envisioned in the 1960s by Lawrence Weed, MD, as a way to transform medical care from diary-like entries into a rigorous and organized system that facilitated diagnosis and treatment [18]. At the time, paper charts lacked easy ways to find the patient's medical conditions and data, and missing something important was a major concern. The problem list system, used today as it was then, is at once comprehensive and flexible; for clinicians working through an active case, especially a patient admitted to the hospital, it allows for a clear way to conceptualize clinical reasoning. Problems may initially be less specific (e.g., "Shortness of breath," "Hypoxia") and later be refined as problems are reorganized with additional data and clinical insight (e.g., "COPD exacerbation due to influenza infection"). Weed's seminal paper even foresaw the use of computers to assist in managing a problem list, addressed the integration of inpatient and outpatient care, advocated for the use of the problem list for preventive health, and included social factors in the examples of problem-oriented medical charting [18].

Fast forward to the present, the electronic health record is now the standard of care. There are newer ways to find information in a chart (e.g., a "search" function rather than flipping through a paper record), amidst a potentially overwhelming amount of information, but the fundamental challenge of maintaining a health record that is complete, yet also useful, remains.

8.3 What Should a Modern Patient-Facing Problem List Include?

There is no consensus as to what constitutes a problem list in an electronic health record [19]. To qualify for US government incentives (e.g., "meaningful use" and subsequent initiatives) through the Centers for Medicare and Medicaid Services,

Table 8.1 Problem list contents

Type of content	Advantages	Disadvantages	Example(s)
Current medical conditions	• The main purpose of the problem list	• Very transient problems may clutter the chart (e.g., URI)	• Hypertension • Diabetes
Past (resolved) medical conditions	• May impact current or future health	• Adds to problem list length • Patients may object to keeping resolved diagnoses in the problem list, especially if potentially stigmatizing	• History of hepatitis C • History of cholecystectomy • History of deep venous thrombosis (DVT)
Risk factors	• May remind clinicians to focus on preventive health and screenings	• Adds to problem list length • Potentially stigmatizing	• Physical inactivity • Family history of breast cancer
Substance use	• May impact current or future health • May remind clinicians to focus on preventive health and screenings	• Adds to problem list length • Potentially stigmatizing, especially if terms such as substance *abuse* are used • Substance use may or may not be problematic	• Opioid use disorder • Injection drug use • Cannabis use • Alcohol use
Social factors	• May emphasize important social determinants of health and increase referrals to community resources	• Adds to problem list length • May be stigmatizing • May overmedicalize social issues	• Homelessness • Food insecurity

clinicians must maintain a problem list of active diagnoses based on the International Classification of Diseases (ICD) or SNOMED CT coding standards [20]. However, there is considerable practice pattern variation regarding what diagnoses clinicians include [3]. Table 8.1 lists possible categories of content for the problem list.

8.3.1   Current Medical Conditions

Most clinicians would agree that a patient's active and chronic medical conditions such as diabetes or hypertension should be included in the problem list. A current condition addressed at an individual visit might be left only as a diagnosis for that encounter and not added to the patient's separate problem list in the electronic health record. For example, a clinician may see a patient for a mild upper respiratory infection—as the patient is expected to recover, the clinician elects not to add *URI* to the patient's problem list.

8.3.2   Past (Resolved) Medical Conditions

Prior medical conditions pose a dilemma for the electronic health record—where should they be located, and what should they be called? There are many options as to how to document past medical conditions, none perfect, all dependent on medical culture and habits of the clinicians using the EHR:

Marking past problems as "resolved": Some electronic health records allow a problem to be marked as "resolved." This method would balance the need to keep a record while not cluttering the current problem list. The issue, however, is whether a clinician will review "resolved" problems. The use of resolved problems may depend on several factors, including whether accessing them requires another step (such as clicking a button, moving to a different tab, and/or changing the default display to visualize "resolved" problems) and what the habits, training, or cultural/organizational expectations are. Notably, in Dr. Weed's original paper, examples are shown in which there are active problems and resolved problems, each in a separate column, on a single page—however not all EHRs have the capability to display the problem list in this manner.

Placing prior medical conditions under "Past Medical History": Similar to a "resolved problems" system, the efficacy of using Past Medical History as a separate part of the electronic health record depends on how easy it is to access and whether clinicians make a practice of accessing it. In addition, this raises the question of what distinguishes Past Medical History and the Problem List in a modern chart. In a traditional history and physical, the past medical history typically contains the patient's current and past conditions; the problem list is then an essential part of the Assessment and Plan and focuses on the current illness. However, outside of an isolated admission note, it is unclear how to distinguish Past Medical History and the Problem list in a modern EHR.

Leaving all past medical conditions in the problem list: Doing so would satisfy the goal of keeping the problem list as comprehensive as possible, in effect being a master list. The risk of this method is that the problem list can become overwhelming to the point of losing utility—if clinicians then stop reading through the problem list, its functionality and purpose are lost.

Deleting past problems completely: This could be considered for a problem that was later diagnosed as a different or more specific condition. For example, for a patient who undergoes an extensive evaluation for dyspnea, but eventually is diagnosed with myasthenia gravis, the initial problem of dyspnea could reasonably be deleted.

In practice, and absent a uniform standard, many clinicians selectively choose which conditions to delete completely, which to keep in the problem list, and which to relegate to resolved problems and/or past medical history. For example, a patient may be treated for a deep venous thrombosis and have an uneventful clinical course. If "DVT" is left as an active problem, it may risk the appearance of an acute DVT or clutter the chart by increasing the length of the problem list. However, if "DVT" is placed elsewhere, there is a risk that a future clinician evaluating the patient for dyspnea may not be aware of this past history and consequently may underestimate the patient's risk for pulmonary embolism. There is no single standard practice—thus, there is an art to maintenance of the problem list.

When it comes to patient-centered language, these decisions can have an impact. Problem lists are often imported into clinical notes and can also be viewed independently by the patient through the electronic health record portal. Patients may be surprised and potentially upset to see a distant problem continually appear on every note. For example, a patient who contracted hepatitis C through a blood transfusion in the 1980s and was subsequently successfully treated may not want to have hepatitis C on their active problem list, concerned that others will assume a history of injection drug use. The clinician, however, may prefer that history remain in the problem list should the patient present to care with elevated liver enzymes. This tension may be especially present for other stigmatized conditions such as substance use, mental health disorders, and obesity.

In the absence of consensus, and with consideration of variations in electronic health records and local practices, we suggest the following:

- If the electronic health record has a "resolved problems" section that is readily viewed and unlikely to be missed: move resolved conditions to that part of the chart.
- If the electronic health record does not have a "resolved problems" section, or if there is a "resolved problems" section but it is structured in such a way that clinicians have a significant likelihood of missing it: include the resolved condition in the usual problem list, and make a note that it is resolved (e.g., *DVT, treated with 3 months of anticoagulation, considered provoked by…—resolved*). Some diagnoses can be coded as "History of …" (e.g., change from *acute DVT* to *History of DVT*).

8.3.3   Risk Factors and Conditions That May Not Be "Problems"

Risk factors and social factors are often included on the problem list if they are deemed to be clinically relevant. To most clinicians, the term "problem list" is a function in and of itself, no longer attached to the original meaning of the word "problem." However, patients often do not share that same understanding.

It is important to consider the implications of documenting risk factors and conditions that might not be actual "problems" (or perceived as problems) in the problem list in the era of the patient-facing electronic health record. Although a risk factor may increase the odds of developing a medical condition and could be important to consider during preventive health visits, patients and clinicians may disagree about whether the risk factor is a "problem" worthy of inclusion on a problem list. For example, although there is a diagnostic code for "Overweight" (E66.3), in the absence of medical complications of elevated body mass index, a patient and clinician may disagree as to whether this constitutes a medical "problem" (see Chap. 5).

Substance use is important to consider. For example, a clinician heeding the recommendations of the US Preventive Services Task Force to screen for unhealthy substance use [21] might document the International Classification of Diseases (ICD)-10 code F12.90 "Use of cannabis" on the problem list. However, the patient may not experience any adverse effects from using cannabis and therefore take issue with this diagnosis included as a "problem." Alcohol is both a food and a substance—while even moderate alcohol use may be a risk factor for multiple conditions, few would add it to a patient's problem list, whereas there is generally more acceptance to adding any amount of cigarette smoking to a problem list. In addition, much of the issue centers not only around terminology (such as avoiding the word *abuse*, see Chap. 10) but also location. If there is a separate location in the electronic health record for substance use, clinicians must make a judgment call regarding when use of a particular substance rises to a threshold to justify inclusion in the Problem List as well.

The documentation of gender identity on the problem list may also be problematic. Diagnostic code F64.0 "Transsexualism" is a stigmatizing and outdated term, but continues to appear on problem lists, pathologizing gender identity. Although gender identity may be relevant to a patient's medical care, it is not a "problem" and is better documented in a separate area of the chart, either as a stand-alone section or in the Social History (see Chaps. 4, 6, and 9) [22]. Diagnoses related to gender may be appropriate to include in the Problem List in certain circumstances. For example, some patients do suffer from gender dysphoria (it should not be assumed that all transgender patients do, however). When providing gender-affirming care, it is helpful to track this information, which may include the use of hormones or surgery, in the Problem List. It is best to work with the patient on finding a term to include in the problem list that the patient is comfortable with and is also medically accurate. ICD-11 has improved terms but has not been rolled out widely in the United States as of this writing [23]. Billing workflows that require gender-affirming prescriptions or referrals to be included under a diagnosis on the problem list further pathologize patients, and workarounds should be developed [24].

Patients receiving preventive therapies may benefit from documentation in the problem list. However, there may be stigmatizing and non-stigmatizing ways to accomplish this. For example, a patient receiving Pre-Exposure Prophylaxis for HIV (PrEP) could have a Problem List diagnosis of Z72.51 ("high-risk heterosexual behavior"), Z72.52 ("high-risk homosexual behavior"), or Z72.53 ("high-risk bisexual behavior"), but these codes are outdated, stigmatizing, and not even particularly medically specific. A more patient-centered code would be "Contact with and (suspected) exposure to HIV" (Z20.6).

If a stigmatizing code must be used, many EHRs have an option to change the display name—if this functionality is available, the clinician can enter a free-text non-stigmatizing term that will be displayed instead. Because the underlying code is still present—even if not seen—it is still best to explain this workaround to the patient (see Chap. 6).

8.3.4   Social Factors as Problems

Most clinicians document psychosocial issues in a separate section of the health record, though they may also include them on the problem list. There are pros and cons to this practice. On the one hand, noting social determinants of health such as Z59.41 "Food insecurity" calls attention to this important issue and may trigger clinicians to connect patients to community resources.

However, viewing food insecurity as a medical problem may also overmedicalize social issues that call for societal fixes, not medical treatment [25]. The impact of viewing social problems as medical problems on patients is unknown. Do patients appreciate their clinician gathering and documenting important social information that clearly impacts their health? Or do patients internalize these problems as personal failures, instead of societal ills?

It is worth noting that nowhere in the problem-oriented electronic health record do we systematically record health-promoting behaviors and strengths. Summarizing a patient in the medical record as a collection of problems to be addressed is a reductionist approach that fails to acknowledge the patient as a human being with medical problems and risk factors but also strengths and resiliencies. Some may argue that adding these additional attributes would clutter an already crowded medical record. However, behavioral health literature suggests that affirming patients and noting strengths are an evidence-based way to enhance patient motivation for healthy behavioral change [26]. If a patient were to view their electronic health record and see health-promoting behaviors listed somewhere in the medical record, perhaps that positive feedback could increase motivation to adopt other healthy behaviors, enhance self-efficacy, and improve health. Future research should assess the impact of strength-based charting in the electronic health record on patient experiences and outcomes.

8.3.5   Alerts and FYIs in the Problem List

There are situations in which it is deemed beneficial that an aspect of a patient's behavior or circumstances be called out in their medical chart in such a way as to alert other healthcare professionals. These alerts may have a range of indications and uses, such as patient safety (e.g., a patient with an unusual allergy, perhaps to something in the waiting room, that most staff would not notice on the patient's allergy list), serious behavioral concerns (e.g., a prior history of threatening behavior toward medical staff), complex multidisciplinary care (e.g., a care plan for a patient admitted to the hospital frequently in order to improve the consistency of their care), or FYIs to other providers about treatments to avoid (e.g., prior problems following a care agreement for controlled substances). In some modern EHRs, there is a separate section of the chart for such alerts that may or may not be visible to the patient, depending on the particular EHR setup. If a clinician chooses to put an alert into a patient's Problem List, they should recognize that patients will now be able to view those alerts; best practices include reconsidering whether the alert is necessary and, if so, remaining factual. For example, if a patient previously did not follow a controlled substance agreement, rather than writing *DO NOT PRESCRIBE CONTROLLED SUBSTANCES* in a patient's problem list, it would be more patient-centered to state the concern factually—*Chronic back pain: previously treated with oxycodone 2014–2016, discontinued after a urine drug screen was reactive for non-prescribed substances. Patient informed that they would not receive chronic opioid therapy from this clinic; now treating with....* Some EHRs allow selected diagnoses to be hidden from a patient—while that may be an option, providers should keep in mind that other clinicians may import the problem list into notes, rendering a previously hidden alert visible; clinicians should also consult with their local compliance staff to ensure that any hidden part of a chart meets criteria for the "information blocking" exception as defined by the Cures Act [27]. As with other themes in this book, even if an alert is not visible to a patient, it is recommended to continue to use best practices of using non-stigmatizing language. Further, when creating alerts, clinicians should be cognizant of potential biases, as there is the potential for discrimination in terms of which patients receive behavioral alerts.

8.4 What Impact Does Viewing the Problem List Have on Patients?

There is an emerging literature on the impact of the patient-facing medical record, but very little has been written on problem lists specifically. In one online survey of patients viewing their problem list, patient attitudes were positive overall [6]. 90.4% of patients rated this exercise as at least somewhat useful. Viewing their problem list evoked happiness in the majority of patients, although some patients reported feeling sad (30.4%), worried (35.7%), or scared (23.8%). Fewer patients reported feeling angry (16.6%) or ashamed (14.3%). Nearly half of patients identified at least one problem missing from the list. 56.1% of patients reported taking at least one action in response to viewing their problem list, including researching a condition on the internet, contacting their healthcare provider, or making plans to change a health behavior. Patients who experienced feeling sad, worried, and scared were most likely to act.

8.5   Language Matters: Best Practices for Management of a Patient-Centered Problem List

Suggested practices for maintaining a patient-centered problem list are shown in Table 8.2.

8.5.1   Consider Renaming or Explaining the "Problem List"

While the term "Problem List" is neutral among healthcare professionals, it may be time to consider alternate nomenclature (e.g., "Health-related issues"). However, it is unlikely that a new consensus term will emerge in the short term—therefore, a short explanatory statement in the patient-facing part of the chart may be helpful (i.e., "The problem list is a medical term that may include medical conditions and other health-related factors that your care team feels are helpful to include in a list. It does not imply that all items listed are 'problems' and we recognize that the term can be confusing.").

Table 8.2 Recommendations for curating an accurate, non-stigmatizing patient-facing problem list

Form follows function	• There is no consensus on which issues belong on a problem list
	• When deciding whether a medical condition, risk factor, or social issue belongs on a problem list, keep in mind the primary function of the problem list as a snapshot view of need-to-know information to enable the treating clinician to provide high-quality medical care
	• When adding any item to the problem list, consider carefully whether it will improve the patient's care
Partner with the patient to ensure accuracy	• Acknowledge that problem lists are often inaccurate and incomplete
	• Convey to your patient that you place a high priority on maintaining an accurate health record
	• Invite patients to review the problem list and point out errors and omissions so they can be corrected
Avoid harmful language	• See Table 8.3 for language to avoid when selecting diagnostic codes for the problem list
	• Invite patients to provide feedback if any language feels uncomfortable or stigmatizing, especially for patients experiencing highly stigmatized conditions such as substance use disorders, obesity, diabetes, chronic pain, and mental health disorders

8.5.2   Use Terms That Are Non-stigmatizing

Stigmas are social constructions that demarcate members of a social group as less worthy and take the form of othering, assigning blame, and invoking danger [14, 28, 29]. Stigmatizing language in the electronic health record has numerous negative impacts on patient care including patients feeling judged after reviewing medical notes [14], which is associated with decreased engagement in healthcare and lower rates of treatment for alcohol use disorder specifically [30, 31]. The electronic health record can transmit bias and stigma between healthcare providers [32–35] and has been shown to affect clinical decision-making about pain management [36]. Patients with substance use disorders, chronic pain, and diabetes are subject to higher rates of stigmatizing language in their medical record [14]. Stigmatizing language is also more frequently found in notes written about Black patients (race identified by EHR data); this has the potential to magnify health inequities associated with racism and undermine trust [14–16, 37]. Despite the known harms of race-based medicine, language in the electronic health record continues to conflate race with biology [38].

Clinicians curating the problem list must choose from available ICD codes, many of which contain harmful language (Table 8.3). Although some recent guidelines on preferred language have been developed in the fields of addiction medicine and diabetes care, most specialties do not have language guides available, and the lexicon is ever-changing [39, 40]. When clinicians are unsure, they can consult their colleagues and their patients whose care is impacted by these choices.

8.5.3   Partnering with Patients to Curate an Accurate, Empowering Problem List

Clinicians should empower their patients to play an active role in curating an accurate, patient-centered problem list. Errors and omissions on the problem list are common [4–6]. Clinicians should openly acknowledge this and ask patients to let them know when mistakes are identified so that they can be promptly corrected. Literature suggests that patient involvement in checking the accuracy of the medical record can improve safety [41–43]. One guideline suggests that clinicians should allow patients to prioritize problems in the order they feel is most important to them [8]. Clinicians should also consider allowing the patient to guide what language is chosen for a certain diagnosis in order to empower patients and lessen stigma. For example, a qualitative study of people with a minoritized gender identity revealed that patients appreciated being asked, "Which diagnosis would you like me to put so that you can get your testosterone covered?" [20].

There will certainly be circumstances in which patients and clinicians disagree on the contents of the problem list. Porter et al. [44] suggested four categories of patient/clinician disputes about the problem list including (1) factual errors (e.g.,

Table 8.3 Diagnoses that contain potentially harmful language

What to avoid	Why	Example(s) of diagnoses and associated codes that contain harmful language	Alternative diagnoses/ codes to consider
Race-based diagnoses	Race is a social construct and is a poor proxy for genetics/biology. Race-based language is stigmatizing and can perpetuate falsehoods associated with race-based medicine	Benign ethnic neutropenia (D70.8)	Typical neutrophil count with Fy(a-b-) status
			Constitutional neutropenia (D70.9)
			Familial benign neutropenia (D70.0)
		Mongolian spot (Q82.8)	Congenital dermal melanocytosis (Q82.8)
Diagnoses easily confused for other conditions	To improve patient understanding of their medical conditions and avoid confusion	Anorexia (R63.0)	Decreased appetite (R63.0) (same code but different label)
Diagnoses that place the blame on the patient	Placing blame on the patient is counterproductive and stigmatizing and may negatively impact the patient/clinician relationship	Abuse of antacids (F55.0)	Gastroesophageal reflux disease (K21.9)—with a description of antacid use
			Milk alkali syndrome (E83.52)
		Failure to demonstrate health literacy (Z55.6)	Problem related to health literacy (Z55.6)
Diagnoses that may confer increased risk for certain conditions but are not medical problems	Medicalizing and pathologizing non-problematic human qualities, identities, and behaviors are stigmatizing	High-risk sexual behavior (Z72.51)	Contact with and (suspected) exposure to HIV (Z20.6)
Other stigmatizing diagnoses and language	Stigma is transmitted through the language used in the medical record and has a wide variety of negative impacts. Patients may lose trust in their clinicians	Opioid abuse (F11.10)	Opioid use disorder (F11.9)

Note: Codes will change depending on what classification system is used—the above are shown as examples

left rather than right knee osteoarthritis), (2) outdated problems that have since resolved (e.g., hypertension that has resolved due to significant weight loss), (3) patient preference to remove actual problems from the problem list (i.e., problem that is accurate and acknowledged by the patient, but the patient does not want

Table 8.4 Questions to guide resolution when the clinician and patient disagree about the contents of the problem list

• I wonder if you have had a chance to review your problem list?
• Were there any things in the problem list that felt inaccurate or uncomfortable?
• What type of change or resolution would you hope to see?
• Is it okay if I explain why we've framed things that way?
• If I cannot change that particular term, are there any other adjustments I could make that might make it more comfortable?

visible on the problem list), and (4) disagreement between patient and provider over whether a problem list item accurately reflects the patient's problem (e.g., a diagnosis of parasite infection by patient versus delusional parasitosis by clinician). While it may be relatively straightforward to resolve disagreements in categories 1 and 2, categories 3 and 4 may be more challenging and ethically fraught. There are no published guidelines on strategies for resolving these disagreements. We recommend that clinicians work through several key questions with patients (Table 8.4) to guide their decision-making.

8.6   Conclusion

The problem list, a snapshot of the patient's most clinically relevant health conditions and issues, can improve clinician efficiency and patient safety and serve as an important communication tool within and between healthcare systems. Clinicians should partner with their patients to agree on a clinically accurate, non-stigmatizing, and respectful approach to the problem list that will balance the needs of both clinicians and patients.

References

1. Simborg DW, Starfield BH, Horn SD, Yourtee SA. Information factors affecting problem follow-up in ambulatory care. Med Care. 1976;14(10):848–56. https://doi.org/10.1097/00005650-197610000-00005.
2. Banerjee ES, Gambler A, Fogleman C. Adding obesity to the problem list increases the rate of providers addressing obesity. Fam Med. 2013;45(9):629–33.
3. Hartung DM, Hunt J, Siemienczuk J, Miller H, Touchette DR. Clinical implications of an accurate problem list on heart failure treatment. J Gen Intern Med. 2005;20(2):143–7. https://doi.org/10.1111/j.1525-1497.2005.40206.x.
4. Holmes C. The problem list beyond meaningful use. Part I: the problems with problem lists. J AHIMA. 2011;82(2):30–3; quiz 34.

5. Wright A, McCoy AB, Hickman TT, et al. Problem list completeness in electronic health records: a multi-site study and assessment of success factors. Int J Med Inform. 2015;84(10):784–90. https://doi.org/10.1016/j.ijmedinf.2015.06.011.
6. Wright A, Feblowitz J, Maloney FL, Henkin S, Ramelson H, Feltman J, Bates DW. Increasing patient engagement: patients' responses to viewing problem lists online. Appl Clin Inform. 2014;5(4):930–42. https://doi.org/10.4338/ACI-2014-07-RA-0057.
7. Wright A, Pang J, Feblowitz JC, Maloney FL, Wilcox AR, Ramelson HZ, Schneider LI, Bates DW. A method and knowledge base for automated inference of patient problems from structured data in an electronic medical record. J Am Med Inform Assoc. 2011;18(6):859–67.
8. Hodge CM, Narus SP. Electronic problem lists: a thematic analysis of a systematic literature review to identify aspects critical to success. J Am Med Inform Assoc. 2018;25(5):603–13. https://doi.org/10.1093/jamia/ocy011.
9. Shah AD, Quinn NJ, Chaudhry A, Sullivan R, Costello J, O'Riordan D, Hoogewerf J, Orton M, Foley L, Feger H, Williams JG. Recording problems and diagnoses in clinical care: developing guidance for healthcare professionals and system designers. BMJ Health Care Inform. 2019;26(1):e100106. https://doi.org/10.1136/bmjhci-2019-100106.
10. Salmi L, Blease C, Hägglund M, Walker J, DesRoches CM. US policy requires immediate release of records to patients. BMJ. 2021;372:n426. https://doi.org/10.1136/bmj.n426.
11. Hägglund M, McMillan B, Whittaker R, Blease C. Patient empowerment through online access to health records. BMJ. 2022;378:e071531. https://doi.org/10.1136/bmj-2022-071531.
12. Walker J, Leveille S, Bell S, Chimowitz H, Dong Z, Elmore JG, Fernandez L, Fossa A, Gerard M, Fitzgerald P, Harcourt K, Jackson S, Payne TH, Perez J, Shucard H, Stametz R, DesRoches C, Delbanco T. OpenNotes after 7 years: patient experiences with ongoing access to their clinicians' outpatient visit notes. J Med Internet Res. 2019;21(5):e13876. https://doi.org/10.2196/13876. Erratum in: J Med Internet Res. 2020;22(4):e18639.
13. Bell SK, Mejilla R, Anselmo M, Darer JD, Elmore JG, Leveille S, Ngo L, Ralston JD, Delbanco T, Walker J. When doctors share visit notes with patients: a study of patient and doctor perceptions of documentation errors, safety opportunities and the patient-doctor relationship. BMJ Qual Saf. 2017;26(4):262–70. https://doi.org/10.1136/bmjqs-2015-004697.
14. Fernández L, Fossa A, Dong Z, et al. Words matter: what do patients find judgmental or offensive in outpatient notes? J Gen Intern Med. 2021;36(9):2571–8. https://doi.org/10.1007/s11606-020-06432-7.
15. Himmelstein G, Bates D, Zhou L. Examination of stigmatizing language in the electronic health record. JAMA Netw Open. 2022;5(1):e2144967. https://doi.org/10.1001/jamanetworkopen.2021.44967.
16. Beach MC, Saha S, Park J, et al. Testimonial injustice: linguistic bias in the medical records of black patients and women. J Gen Intern Med. 2021;36(6):1708–14. https://doi.org/10.1007/s11606-021-06682-z.
17. Sun M, Oliwa T, Peek ME, Tung EL. Negative patient descriptors: documenting racial bias in the electronic health record. Health Aff (Millwood). 2022;41(2):203–11.
18. Weed LL. Medical records that guide and teach. N Engl J Med. 1968;278(11):593–600. https://doi.org/10.1056/NEJM196803142781105.
19. Holmes C, Brown M, Hilaire DS, Wright A. Healthcare provider attitudes towards the problem list in an electronic health record: a mixed-methods qualitative study. BMC Med Inform Decis Mak. 2012;12:127. https://doi.org/10.1186/1472-6947-12-127.
20. Office of the National Coordinator for Health Information Technology (ONC), Department of Health and Human Services. Health information technology: initial set of standards, implementation specifications, and certification criteria for electronic health record technology. Final rule. Fed Regist. 2010;75(144):44589–654.

21. Preventive Services Task Force US, Krist AH, Davidson KW, et al. Screening for unhealthy drug use: US Preventive Services Task Force recommendation statement. JAMA. 2020;323(22):2301–9. https://doi.org/10.1001/jama.2020.8020.
22. Kronk CA, Everhart AR, Ashley F, Thompson HM, Schall TE, Goetz TG, Hiatt L, Derrick Z, Queen R, Ram A, Guthman EM, Danforth OM, Lett E, Potter E, Sun SED, Marshall Z, Karnoski R. Transgender data collection in the electronic health record: current concepts and issues. J Am Med Inform Assoc. 2022;29(2):271–84. https://doi.org/10.1093/jamia/ocab136.
23. World Health Organization. Gender incongruence and transgender health in the ICD. https://www.who.int/standards/classifications/frequently-asked-questions/gender-incongruence-and-transgender-health-in-the-icd. Accessed 20 Mar 2023.
24. Alpert AB, Mehringer JE, Orta SJ, et al. Experiences of transgender people reviewing their electronic health records, a qualitative study. J Gen Intern Med. 2023;38(4):970–7. https://doi.org/10.1007/s11606-022-07671-6.
25. Lantz PM. The medicalization of population health: who will stay upstream? Milbank Q. 2019;97(1):36–9. https://doi.org/10.1111/1468-0009.12363.
26. Bischof G, Bischof A, Rumpf HJ. Motivational interviewing: an evidence-based approach for use in medical practice. Dtsch Arztebl Int. 2021;118(7):109–15. https://doi.org/10.3238/arztebl.m2021.0014.
27. The Office of the National Coordinator for Health Information Technology. Cures act final rule: information blocking exceptions (HealthIt.gov). https://www.healthit.gov/sites/default/files/2022-07/InformationBlockingExceptions.pdf. Accessed 27 May 2023.
28. Goffman E. Stigma: notes on the management of spoiled identity. Englewood Cliffs, NJ: Prentice-Hall; 1963.
29. Smith RA. Language of the lost: an explication of stigma communication. Commun Theory. 2007;17(4):462–85. https://doi.org/10.1111/j.1468-2885.2007.00307.x.
30. Puhl R, Peterson JL, Luedicke J. Motivating or stigmatizing? Public perceptions of weight-related language used by health providers. Int J Obes (Lond). 2013;37(4):612–9.
31. Keyes KM, Hatzenbuehler ML, McLaughlin KA, et al. Stigma and treatment for alcohol disorders in the United States. Am J Epidemiol. 2010;172(12):1364–72. https://doi.org/10.1093/aje/kwq304.
32. Kelly JF, Westerhoff CM. Does it matter how we refer to individuals with substance-related conditions? A randomized study of two commonly used terms. Int J Drug Policy. 2010;21(3):202–7. https://doi.org/10.1016/j.drugpo.2009.10.010.
33. Ashford RD, Brown AM, McDaniel J, Curtis B. Biased labels: an experimental study of language and stigma among individuals in recovery and health professionals. Subst Use Misuse. 2019;54(8):1376–84. https://doi.org/10.1080/10826084.2019.1581221.
34. Andraka-Christou B, Capone MJ. A qualitative study comparing physician-reported barriers to treating addiction using buprenorphine and extended-release naltrexone in U.S. office-based practices. Int J Drug Policy. 2018;54:9–17. https://doi.org/10.1016/j.drugpo.2017.11.021.
35. Ashford RD, Brown AM, Curtis B. "Abusing addiction": our language still isn't good enough. Alcohol Treat Q. 2019;37(2):257–72. https://doi.org/10.1080/07347324.2018.1513777.
36. Goddu AP, O'Conor KJ, Lanzkron S, et al. Do words matter? Stigmatizing language and the transmission of bias in the medical record. J Gen Intern Med. 2018;33(5):685–91. https://doi.org/10.1007/s11606-017-4289-2.
37. Hatzenbuehler ML, Phelan JC, Link BG. Stigma as a fundamental cause of population health inequalities. Am J Public Health. 2013;103(5):813–21.
38. Cerdeña JP, Plaisime MV, Tsai J. From race-based to race-conscious medicine: how anti-racist uprisings call us to act. Lancet. 2020;396(10257):1125–8. https://doi.org/10.1016/S0140-6736(20)32076-6.
39. Kelly JF, Saitz R, Wakeman S. Language, substance use disorders, and policy: the need to reach consensus on an "addiction-ary". Alcohol Treat Q. 2016;34(1):116–23. https://doi.org/10.1080/07347324.2016.1113103.

40. Dickinson JK, Guzman SJ, Maryniuk MD, et al. The use of language in diabetes care and education. Diabetes Care. 2017;40(12):1790–9. https://doi.org/10.2337/dci17-0041.
41. Blease CR, Bell SK. Patients as diagnostic collaborators: sharing visit notes to promote accuracy and safety. Diagnosis (Berl). 2019;6(3):213–21. https://doi.org/10.1515/dx-2018-0106.
42. Neves AL, Freise L, Laranjo L, Carter AW, Darzi A, Mayer E. Impact of providing patients access to electronic health records on quality and safety of care: a systematic review and meta-analysis. BMJ Qual Saf. 2020;29:1019–32. https://doi.org/10.1136/bmjqs-2019-010581.
43. National Academies of Sciences, Engineering, and Medicine. Improving diagnosis in health care. 2015. https://www.nap.edu/catalog/21794/improving-diagnosis-in-health-care.
44. Porter AS, O'Callaghan J, Englund KA, Lorenz RR, Kodish E. Problems with the problem list: challenges of transparency in an era of patient curation. J Am Med Inform Assoc. 2020;27(6):981–4. https://doi.org/10.1093/jamia/ocaa040.

Chapter 9
The Social History

Rebecca D. Ellis and Renata Thronson

9.1 Introduction

The social history is an essential part of the medical evaluation. Exploring social determinants of health and health-related behaviors is critical to patient care. Historically, much attention has been paid within medical education on how to gather components of the social history in a way that is culturally and individually sensitive. Providers are often educated, for example, on inclusive sexual history taking through open-ended communication practices and increased awareness of the spectrum of gender identity and sexual orientation. Little guidance exists, however, on how to document that history in a way that promotes patient consideration and inclusion. Furthermore, language that may be stigmatizing or judgmental to patients may crop up more frequently in documentation of the social history, as the relevant information—occupation, racial and ethnic identity, religion, substance use, and sexual practices, among other topics—may create more opportunities for bias and discrimination. Nevertheless, documenting the social history offers unique opportunities for patient engagement and authorship in their medical care, since patients' individual social environments and behaviors are highly linked with health outcomes.

In this chapter, we will explore how Open Notes promote patient engagement with health components belonging to the social history. We will then examine how common documentation practices might pose potential for patient harm and, conversely, explore methods for cultivating humanistic, patient-centered language in the medical record. Next, we will highlight important considerations regarding

R. D. Ellis · R. Thronson (✉)
Division of General Internal Medicine, Department of Medicine, University of Washington, Seattle, WA, USA
e-mail: ellisrd@uw.edu; lrenata@uw.edu

© The Author(s), under exclusive license to Springer Nature Switzerland AG 2023
C. J. Wong, S. L. Jackson (eds.), *The Patient-Centered Approach to Medical Note-Writing*, https://doi.org/10.1007/978-3-031-43633-8_9

confidentiality within the electronic medical record. Lastly, we will explore the virtues of automated entry and possibilities for patient authorship in the social history.

The aim of this chapter is not to define the components of a social history, but rather to provide best practices for choosing language for documentation that is most patient-centered. Our goal is to provide a framework for documenting the social history in a way that minimizes physical and psychological harm to patients and empowers patients in their healthcare journey.

9.2   Merits of Open Notes and Opportunities for Patient Engagement

In accordance with the 21st Century Cures Act of 2016, patients are intended rapid, free, and complete access to their medical record including clinical notes and personal health information. As well documented elsewhere in this book, open access to patient charts has demonstrated widespread benefits—in particular, improving patient-doctor communication, promoting patient education, and heightening patient engagement with medical care [1]. The concept of "open notes" emphasizes that documentation should be geared towards patients as much as it is towards fellow healthcare professionals. At a glance, increasing patient readership might seem burdensome to providers; various qualitative studies have revealed apprehensions among providers about increased time devoted to crafting documentation easily understood by patients, censoring, and even misrepresenting medical decision-making for fear of troubling patients, among other concerns [2–4]. The social history, however, lends itself easily to patient-centered documentation because it includes psychosocial information that is uniquely free from clinical content and therefore medical jargon. The social history is perhaps the area in medical care where patients can contribute the most authorship in their healthcare, since it pertains to personal health-related behaviors and social determinants of health.

9.3   Components of the Social History

There is no universal definition of what features belong to the social history. Many social history frameworks have been put forward, which comprise a variety of subjects, including race, ethnicity, marital status, children, diet, exercise, substance use, environmental exposures, living situation, religion, employment, military service, and home safety [5]. In general, the social history aims to capture an individual's interaction with society by describing their behaviors, relationships, and environmental circumstances. There is certainly overlap between the medical history and social history, as items commonly included in the social history—for example, homelessness and tobacco—can often be considered medical conditions in their own right.

One study found that the elements most commonly included in the social history are alcohol use, tobacco use, drug use, family descriptions, living situation and residence, marital status, and occupation [5]. Behforouz et al. propose a thoughtful reimagining of the Social History with the goal of discovering an individual's personal and contextual identity over and above mere "habits" and facts. They recommend the following six social history topics: individual characteristics, life circumstances, emotional health, perceptions of healthcare, health-related behaviors, and access to and utilization of healthcare [6]. These categories were written with the patient's perspective in mind and therefore lend themselves to patient-centered language. They are also highly adaptable to the clinical setting and population at hand. Providers might consider adopting these classifications as patient-facing headings when documenting the social history.

It is important to note that what constitutes an adequate social history may be unique to the particular population that is being served. For instance, a primary care clinic that serves patients belonging primarily to a geriatric population may highlight features of a social history pertaining to older adults, such as caregivers and social support, activities of daily living, and advanced care planning. Meanwhile, a primary care clinic housed in a treatment center for substance use disorders may prioritize different areas within the social history, such as access to safe transportation and housing, employment, and drug and alcohol use.

It is worth noting that some topics typical of the social history can be so complex that they may be worthy of assessment and documentation as their own category outside of the social history. For example, exploring a patient's exercise habits may involve questions about access to safe spaces for exercise, available time outside of work for exercise, and financial concerns related to exercise. Similarly, exploring a patient's nutrition might involve assessing a patient's access to healthy foods, dietary restrictions, and history of disordered eating behaviors.

9.4   Social History Chart Documentation: Obtaining and Structuring Data in the Electronic Health Record (EHR)

Social history may be obtained by direct interview with a patient by a healthcare professional or through patient self-report via the use of questionnaires and surveys. For many providers, electronic health records offer increasing opportunities for standardized entries, such as drop-down menus and multiple-choice selections. EHRs with standardized data entry fields that use patient-centered language may minimize opportunities for bias compared to narrative, free-text documentation of the social history. Neutral and inclusive language in data selections and category names can normalize documentation of a patient's social history as well as the process of obtaining it.

It is increasingly common for patients to contribute information that is relevant to the social history through paper questionnaires or directly into the EHR through secure patient portals. It may be more comfortable and accurate for patients to share sensitive information independently rather than in verbal conversation with their provider. The transition from provider-controlled to patient-directed documentation is an opportunity to cultivate patient autonomy and psychological safety. Best practices for EHR design include provider and patient input to ensure that standardized data fields contain patient-centered language and information that is considered important to both patients and providers.

There is no consensus on how to organize social history data in a medical note. It might be reasonable to document all of the social history elements as free text in paragraph form or divide the social history under subcategories (e.g., living environment, sexual history, etc.). If headings are used, they should be patient-centered, as outdated or inaccurate headings can be harmful to patients. For example, *Sexual Preference* as a heading is an inappropriate term for sexual orientation. In addition, order of headings should be standardized in the EHR in a way that is clear and promotes psychological safety. People might feel more comfortable, for instance, disclosing and reading about their diet and exercise habits before their sexual practices (although there may certainly be exceptions). Data should be collected and organized with these considerations in mind.

Social history data is usually stored in an area of the EHR that is separate from progress note writing. It is crucial that this information be verified before transferring it into a medical note. It is not uncommon for outdated social history data to be transferred accidentally into the medical note, and this data should therefore be reviewed and updated regularly. In addition, the note writer should check imported data for patient-centered language. Language is continually evolving, and EHR fields may not be up to date with contemporary or correct terminology. For example, an EHR questionnaire may list "illicit drugs," whereas the clinician might avoid this term (see Chap. 10) when writing the note free-text.

9.5   Open Notes and Potential for Harm

Unfortunately, it is not uncommon for patients to report feeling judged or offended by something they have read in their medical record. Phrasing taught to medical professionals—either explicitly in training or through the hidden curriculum—is unfortunately ripe with opportunity for harm, especially when used to document the social history. Férnandez et al. identified three major types of injury we ought to consider when writing in the medical record: misrepresentation, labeling, and disrespect [7]. Patients can be offended when medical notes include inaccuracies and medical decision-making not shared with the patient during the visit. Second, patients can experience stigma and discrimination when they are or feel labeled by descriptors, identifiers, or pejorative terms. Third, patients can feel disrespected by many things they might read in the medical record; this reaction is specifically triggered by language that is dismissive or undervalues their perspective. These are all important areas worth considering when creating notes that are patient-centered, but it is in these second and third domains that we will spend most of our time exploring in the remainder of this chapter.

9.6   Language to Adopt and Habits to Avoid in Documenting the Social History

How do we create a more humanistic approach to documentation that minimizes harm towards patients and promotes patient engagement? Several guides exist on preferred language in medical documentation, many of which have been spearheaded by patient advocacy groups and are informed by the lived experience of patients.

Healy et al. [8] outline several important features of patient-centered language. Perhaps the most critical feature is person-first language, which refers to separating a condition from the individual instead of defining the person by their condition. *A person experiencing homelessness* is an example of a person-first description, whereas *homeless person* is not. A second feature is inclusive language, which seeks to avoid categories, terms, or expressions that exclude particular groups or frame them as "other." This involves deliberately choosing words that may capture a wide set of experiences or identities and avoids assumptions. For example, *relationship status* is a more inclusive descriptor than *marital status*, as it acknowledges the variety of relationships that patients may experience rather than simply *married/single*.

A key feature of patient-centered language is avoiding weaponizing quotations since, as has been well-documented throughout this book, they may devalue and discredit the patient experience (see Chaps. 3 and 7). Though frequently used to recite patient's own words, quotations can cast skepticism or discredit. Consider the statements *the patient states he drinks 'socially'* and *the patient uses condoms 'most of the time'*. The use of quotation marks here seems to call into question the patient's report and, if read by a patient, might feel insulting—as though their provider does not trust them or is making fun of them. Of course, there are times in which quotation marks might add value by purposefully highlighting a patient's perspective, for example, during a goals-of-care discussion or mental health evaluation. We recommend providers to ask themselves if their use of quotation marks is truly necessary to convey meaning or whether it is gratuitous or harmful.

Furthermore, it is crucial that providers eliminate pejorative and judgmental terminology from their documentation that may insult and harm patients. When in doubt, it is almost always appropriate to use the words or phrases that patients themselves use to convey their experience, as paraphrasing or rewriting may open the door to potential harmful language. For example, perhaps a patient says they walk once a week, and the provider writes *the patient does little exercise* or *the patient is not an exerciser.* Paraphrasing in this way provides a poor and perhaps insulting summation of this person's exercise habits. We recommend providers to ask themselves frequently: "Does what I've written assign blame?," and "Can I be more specific?" Our language should be nonjudgmental, and it should also be adequately descriptive, both for our colleagues and for our patients. Consider the following descriptions: *the patient is addicted to illicit drug*s and *the patient injects heroin daily.* The second description is both clearer and more supportive by virtue of being more specific. As a general rule, making an effort to describe specific experiences rather than generalizing behaviors of patients minimizes the opportunity for harmful biases and unfair value judgments. Certainly, it would be impractical for a provider to fully describe a patient's life experience. However, small moves towards specificity and completeness can make a meaningful difference in the way of compassionate representation.

It is through these principles that we will explore how to document common items of the social history in a patient-centered fashion. This list is by no means exhaustive, but serves to represent areas that are frequently encountered in the social history (Table 9.1).

9.6.1 Race and Ethnicity

It is not recommended to include race or ethnic identifiers in the "one-liner" (Chap. 7) or physical exam (Chap. 12). The Social History section, however, is an appropriate place to document a patient's racial and ethnic identification. If documented from an interview, race and ethnicity should be part of a larger discussion of identity and should be explored in an open-ended manner. A patient's identification should almost always be documented verbatim and not approximated or automatically recategorized. For example, if a patient identifies as Black, the note writer should not write African American, or if the patient identifies as Taiwanese American, the note writer should not write Asian. If data is imported or reviewed from other sources (questionnaires, other parts of the chart), it should be verified, as race and ethnicity are often collected using the 1997 Office of Management and Budget standards, which are limited to five races and two ethnicities [9], or other questionnaires with inadequate or few choices. Patients might feel forced to choose an option that they do not actually identify with or select "Other" if they do not find appropriate options. The limitations of having too few options were highlighted by the US Census Bureau's research finding that "Other" became the third-largest racial group in the 2010 Census [10]. (See Chap. 4 for further discussion of race and ethnicity.)

Table 9.1 Examples of social history language recommendations

Language principle	Harmful phrasing	Suggested alternative
Choose person-first language: Put the patient before the condition or behavior	*Drug addict; alcoholic*	*Person with a history of substance use or alcohol use disorder*
	Tobacco user	*Person with a history of tobacco use*
	Homeless person	*Person who is experiencing homelessness*
	Uninsured person	*Person without health insurance*
Eliminate pejorative terms: Use patient-preferred and specific terminology	*Illegal immigrant, foreigner, alien*	*… has undocumented status … immigrated from ___ … refugee (if appropriate) … is seeking asylum (if appropriate)*
	Financially unstable	*Financial insecurity, difficulty making ends meet*
	Domestic violence	*Intimate partner violence*
	Rape victim	*Person who has experienced sexual assault or rape*
	Convict, prisoner	*Person experiencing incarceration*
	Relapse	*Return to use*
	Sober	*In remission/recovery from substance use*
	Social drinker	*Drinks 2 alcoholic beverages per week*
Eliminate judgment: Describe observed behaviors or reported experiences without judgment Omit commentary	*Risky sex* *Unprotected sex*	Describe behavior: *e.g., Condomless anal receptive sex, vaginal sex with a male partner, without contraceptive methods*
	Patient is drug seeking	*The patient is experiencing cravings for opioids*
	Patient is a frequent flyer	Describe recent healthcare without label or commentary: e.g., *patient was admitted 3 months ago and 1 month ago for a similar presentation*
	Poor health literacy	*Difficulty accessing care due to English as second language, difficulty reading medical instructions, etc.*

(continued)

Table 9.1 (continued)

Language principle	Harmful phrasing	Suggested alternative

Minimize quotations:
  Remove quotations that may cast doubt or skepticism
  Incorporate other indications that a patient is speaking or sharing perspective
	The patient is "cutting back on tobacco"	*The patient is cutting back on tobacco*

	The patient "always uses condoms"	*The patient uses barrier protection consistently*
	The patient declined home health because "I won't let anyone in my house because the government is out to get me"	*The patient declined home health because he does not want to let anyone into his house as he worries the government is out to get him*
Utilize the patient's own words: Avoid paraphrasing or summarizing to minimize risk of misrepresentation	*The patient is monogamous*	*The patient has one sexual partner, their spouse*

9.6.2 Gender

Gender information is often stored in multiple locations in the EHR. In some EHRs there is a separate section where patient-centered data can be inputted, including gender identity and pronouns. It is critical for the provider to verify the person's gender identity and pronouns before they are automatically transmitted into the document to avoid including outdated or incorrect information. If documented in social history, a patient's gender should be noted as *gender* or *gender identity*, not *gender preference*—as this is an outdated term and may be harmful to patients. Gender identity and sex assigned at birth are usually not necessary to be noted in one-liners or other identifying statements (see Chap. 7), but they may be appropriate to include in a medical note if a visit is specifically dedicated towards gender care. (See Chap. 4 for further discussion of gender.)

9.6.3 Marital Status and Family Structure

There are several ways in which documentation of marital status and family structure has excluded individuals and groups that do not conform to traditional social conventions, namely, the nuclear family and heterosexual marriages. It is crucial that providers choose inclusive language in documentation of marital status and family structure that minimizes assumptions and acknowledges the wide range of human experience. For example, a patient with serious illness may belong to a polyamorous relationship with multiple people; open discussion and documentation of this patient's experience are crucial to understanding the support system and hierarchy of surrogate decision-makers that are unique to them. In addition, providers should use correct and inclusive pronouns when referring to a patient's family members, romantic partners, and friends. If unknown, providers should choose gender-neutral pronouns (e.g., *they/them*). Accordingly, providers should utilize neutral or general descriptors (e.g., words such as *significant other* or *partner* instead of *girlfriend* or *wife*) when documenting relationships in order to minimize assumptions and promote truthfulness, especially when there is uncertainty.

9.6.4 Tobacco, Alcohol, and Other Substances

In documentation of tobacco, alcohol, and substance use, it is especially crucial to utilize person-first language and avoid pejorative terminology. *Alcoholic* and *smoker* suggest that the substance use is an inherent part of the person and therefore does not reflect person-first language. *The patient smokes a half-pack per day of cigarettes*, *the patient has alcohol use disorder*, and *a person who uses drugs* are, on the other hand, examples of person-first language. When describing drug use, words such as *relapse* and *addict* connote judgment; *return to use* and *substance use disorder* are more supportive alternatives. When in doubt, it is better to simply describe the behavior of the person, in order to minimize opportunity for judgment and labeling.

In some cases, a patient may self-identify as an addict or an alcoholic as a way to understand their condition and be able to take the necessary steps to address it—in those cases this self-identification can be documented (e.g., *Patient identifies as an alcoholic and is in recovery. They are now 300 days from their last drink*). It is through use of the patient's own language that the clinician honors the patient's experience and treats them as a whole person. Exploration with the patient is recommended to distinguish if the patient's use of specific terminology is affirming versus self-stigmatizing (Chap. 10), as it is not uncommon for patients to internalize societal condemnation through the use of these terms (e.g., *addict*, *alcoholic*, etc.) in a way that may be disempowering.

For other substances, terms such as *abuse*, *recreational drugs*, *illicit drugs*, and *illegal drugs* should be avoided, for the following reasons. The term *abuse* connotes a risky or dangerous behavior and may cast undue blame on a patient, regardless of whether or not they have a substance use disorder. States have varying laws regarding drug use, and words such as *illicit* or *illegal* may be incorrect in addition to casting judgment. Moreover, it would be inappropriate to describe drug use that may be intended for therapeutic effect (e.g. marijuana) as recreational. Lastly, for patients living with addiction, there may, in fact, be no recreational aspect to their use. Overall, these terms can easily misrepresent the lived experience and behaviors of patients and should therefore be avoided unless explicitly used by the patient. See Chap. 10 for further discussion of substance use.

9.6.5 Sexual Health

Similarly, in documentation of the sexual history, it is critical that providers provide clear representation of the patient's behaviors without attributing judgment or pejorative terminology. For example, the phrases *risky sexual behaviors* and *unprotected sex* are both criticizing and vague. Although *unprotected sex* is often thought to describe condomless sex, this association cannot be taken for granted. It is worth emphasizing to ourselves and our patients that interventions to prevent pregnancy and sexually transmitted infections (STIs) are not one and the same. On top of that, the word *protection* might imply that the avoided outcome (e.g., STIs, pregnancy) is indecent or shameful. Instead, we recommend simply recording types of sex practiced, pharmacologic and barrier methods utilized to prevent STIs, and forms of contraception applied. It is through accurate and clear documentation that sexual health can be recorded in a patient-centered way.

9.6.6 Housing Status

There are many terms for housing status, including homeless, houseless, unhoused/housed, undomiciled/domiciled, unstably housed, or having unstable housing. It is good practice to discuss terminology with an individual patient to identify language that best represents the patient's experience. As described in the previous sections, certain terms such as *homeless*, though frequently used, may cause harm due to labeling if not reviewed with the patient prior to documentation. An individual who resides in a shelter may indeed have a place they perceive as home, and the word *homeless* may be hurtful to read in the chart. To be *housed* can refer to any type of shelter or living accommodation and may not fully capture the reality of an individual patient. It is worth noting that some advocates embrace the term *homeless* for advocacy and outreach (and is often required for tracking or funding purposes), despite it being a challenging and charged term for many. With these considerations in mind, it is ideal for providers to explicitly describe the living circumstances of the patient without ascribing a particular label or interpretation. Appropriate examples include the following: *the patient lives in an apartment downtown* or *lives in their van and sometimes stays with a friend* or *works during the day and sleeps on the street at night*. Again, it is recommended that providers prioritize person-first language (e.g., *person who lives in a shelter*) instead of labeling a patient by their lack of housing (e.g., *homeless person*).

9.6.7 Occupation and Finances

Descriptions such as *unemployed* or *financially unstable* may not effectively capture the life circumstances of the patient and, moreover, assign fault to the individual when often there are complex personal and societal forces at play. Rather, describing the patient's situation in plain language may be more useful by promoting clarity and minimizing potential for insult, e.g., *The patient does not currently have a job while caring for their mother who is on hospice*, or *The patient is experiencing difficulty paying rent on time*. Outdated terms that may connote judgment such as *homemaker* and *breadwinner* should be avoided.

9.6.8 Carceral Status

A patient's incarceration history should be discussed and documented with care. One study found that men who had been recently released from prison had high rates of self-reported discrimination from healthcare workers [11]. Ideally, all patients should be screened for history of incarceration. By only asking patients suspected of having an incarceration history, providers will not only invite harmful biases into their care of particular patients but will also neglect individuals who have been incarcerated and are vulnerable to important diseases and hardships [12]. A history of incarceration is an important social determinant of health, as incarceration is associated with a higher burden of chronic diseases [13]. Moreover, there are increased rates of morbidity and mortality in the transition period after release from incarceration, attributed to gaps in healthcare coverage and social support [14].

It is almost never appropriate to inquire or document a patient's reason for incarceration, as it is very likely irrelevant to the patient's care and encourages bias from future providers. Doing so may invite undue speculation, substandard care, and, potentially, objection to treatment. Furthermore, an individual's reason for incarceration may not adequately reflect the reality of their actions or their circumstances—a person who is incarcerated may be in jail awaiting trial or in prison falsely convicted. Even if the reason for a patient's incarceration is revealed, it should generally not be documented in the chart, as this information may compromise their opportunity for equitable care from future providers.

9.6.9 Immigration Status

Like other socially and politically charged areas of the social history, immigration status should be discussed and documented with care. Some patients who immigrate, particularly refugees, have experienced trauma and unique exposures that may make them vulnerable to certain physical and mental conditions. Patients who are undocumented or refugees may hesitate to seek care, for fear of exposure, language and cultural barriers, and financial burdens, among other concerns. Efforts should be made by providers to honor these concerns and promote the patient's sense of safety, both through culturally appropriate communication and discreet documentation. Though it may be important to gather an immigration history to highlight relevant medical exposures or risk factors, it is critical that providers document this information with caution and only to the extent that it is relevant to the patient's care. In addition, there are terms that may cause harm, and that should be avoided, including *illegal immigrant*, *alien*, and *foreigner*.

9.6.10 Language Preference or Proficiency

As discussed in Chap. 7, language preference or proficiency is generally not recommended in one-liners or summative statements but might be noted if an interpreter is used. The social history section is an appropriate place to document more richly a patient's language history. Patients may speak multiple languages, with varying degrees of proficiency have potential differences between written and oral communication; and have different preferences for what language to use in the healthcare setting.

9.7 Confidentiality and Keeping Personal Health Information Safe

It is worth exploring the notion of confidentiality as it pertains to increasing patient access to medical records. Confidentiality is critical to establishing trust and a safe environment for utilizing healthcare. Patients might be surprised, however, to find information in the medical chart that they thought was shared privately with their provider. There may be misunderstanding between the provider and the patient on what is considered truly confidential. Importantly, there is potential for disagreement about whether documenting information in the chart represents a breach of this confidentiality, insofar as other providers and proxy users of the patient-facing electronic health record have access to that information. This issue is particularly salient among more sensitive topics typically found in the social history.

Much like any other element of patient care, it is critical that providers clearly discuss the process and implications of medical documentation to establish a shared mental model of confidentiality. It is only through clear communication that patients can access and grant proxy access to their medical records in a safe, informed way. Personal health information is protected in accordance with the *Standards for Privacy of Individually Identifiable Health Information* ("Privacy Rule") under the Health Insurance Portability and Accountability Act (HIPAA). Though these standards are complex patients should be informed at the time of registering for healthcare, and again if they register with an electronic health record's patient portal, that health information documented in the medical chart is highly protected and, at the same time, accessible to other healthcare professionals to permit effective healthcare delivery. Providers may need to review these standards with their patients.

It is common for patients to share electronic health information and access with friends or family members. It is therefore crucial for providers to inquire about who else besides their patient can access their medical record. Documenting certain elements of the social history may have important implications for patients should this information be read by other parties. In the worst-case scenario, significant harm is possible: for example, documenting intimate partner violence may put a patient at further risk if their partner has access to the medical record. Or patients may simply not want certain information visible to friends or family members who may have access to their medical record. A patient-provider discussion of confidentiality in the medical record should establish the scope of the social history documentation. Providers should make clear that it may not be possible for certain aspects of the EHR to be guarded from access on the patient portal. Patients should be aware that any person accessing the medical record will likely be able to see it in its entirety, for this may inform if they choose to grant proxy access.

9.8   Conclusion

In conclusion, there are several important themes that have emerged in this chapter and may point us towards more humanistic, patient-centered documentation. In general, when documenting the social history, it is crucial that providers choose person-first language, adopt patient-preferred terminology, and, when in doubt, emphasize the patient's own words without the use of weaponizing quotations. In addition, providers should minimize criticism and commentary by describing specifically observed behaviors and reported experiences of patients.

Perhaps more important than familiarizing oneself with a list of documentation "dos and don'ts" is cultivating an attitude towards growth—that is, an appreciation that our words have meaning and a willingness to revise and adapt our language in a way that meets our patients' needs. The authors of this chapter acknowledge that there are words and phrases we recommend today that we may abandon tomorrow. Remaining open to feedback and committing to improvement are the most important steps we can take to making our documentation more accessible and less biased. We should continue to shape our practices in a way that prioritizes the health and safety of those patients who are marginalized or oppressed. Their feedback should be invited and their voices incorporated into medical documentation. Our patients are our greatest guide towards a more inclusive, collaborative, and humanistic practice.

References

1. Delbanco T, Walker J, Darer JD, et al. Open notes: doctors and patients signing on. Ann Intern Med. 2010;153(2):121–5. https://doi.org/10.7326/0003-4819-153-2-201007200-00008.
2. Alpert JM, Morris BB, Thomson MD, Matin K, Sabo RT, Brown RF. Patient access to clinical notes in oncology: a mixed method analysis of oncologists' attitudes and linguistic characteristics towards notes. Patient Educ Couns. 2019;102(10):1917–24. https://doi.org/10.1016/j.pec.2019.05.008.
3. Delbanco T, Walker J, Bell SK, et al. Inviting patients to read their doctors' notes: a quasi-experimental study and a look ahead. Ann Intern Med. 2012;157(7):461–70. https://doi.org/10.7326/0003-4819-157-7-201210020-00002.
4. Crotty BH, et al. Open notes in teaching clinics: a multisite survey of residents to identify anticipated attitudes and guidance for programs. J Grad Med Educ. 2018;10(3):292–300. https://doi.org/10.4300/jgme-d-17-00486.1.
5. Chen ES, Manaktala S, Sarkar IN, Melton GB. A multi-site content analysis of social history information in clinical notes. AMIA Annu Symp Proc. 2011;2011:227–36.
6. Behforouz HL, Drain PK, Rhatigan JJ. Rethinking the social history. N Engl J Med. 2014;371(14):1277–9. https://doi.org/10.1056/NEJMp1404846.
7. Fernández L, Fossa A, Dong Z, et al. Words matter: what do patients find judgmental or offensive in outpatient notes? J Gen Intern Med. 2021;36(9):2571–8. https://doi.org/10.1007/s11606-020-06432-7.
8. Healy M, Richard A, Kidia K. How to Reduce Stigma and Bias in Clinical Communication: a Narrative Review. J Gen Intern Med. 2022;37(10):2533–2540. https://doi.org/10.1007/s11606-022-07609-y. Epub 2022 May 6. PMID: 35524034; PMCID: PMC9360372.
9. Office of Management and Budget. Revisions to the standards for the classification of federal data on race and ethnicity. Fed Regist. 1997;62(210):58782–90. https://www.govinfo.gov/content/pkg/FR-1997-10-30/pdf/97-28653.pdf. Accessed 13 Feb 2023.
10. Mathews K, Phelan J, Jones NA, Konya S, Marks R, Pratt BM, Coombs J, Bentley M. 2015 National Content Test. Race and ethnicity analysis report. Issued 28 Feb 2017. https://www2.census.gov/programs-surveys/decennial/2020/program-management/final-analysis-reports/2015nct-race-ethnicity-analysis.pdf. Accessed 13 Feb 2023.
11. Frank JW, Wang EA, Nunez-Smith M, et al. Discrimination based on criminal record and healthcare utilization among men recently released from prison: a descriptive study. Health Justice. 2014;2:6. https://doi.org/10.1186/2194-7899-2-6.
12. Sue K. How to talk with patients about incarceration and health. AMA J Ethics. 2017;19(9):885–93. https://doi.org/10.1001/journalofethics.2017.19.9.ecas2-1709.
13. Kendig NE, Butkus R, Mathew S, Hilden D, Health and Public Policy Committee of the American College of Physicians. Health care during incarceration: a policy position paper from the American college of physicians. Ann Intern Med. 2022;175(12):1742–5. https://doi.org/10.7326/M22-2370.
14. Binswanger IA, Stern MF, Deyo RA, et al. Release from prison—a high risk of death for former inmates [published correction appears in N Engl J Med. 2007 Feb 1;356(5):536]. N Engl J Med. 2007;356(2):157–65. https://doi.org/10.1056/NEJMsa064115.

Chapter 10
Substance Use and Substance Use Disorders

Russell Berg, Jocelyn James, and Jared W. Klein

10.1   Introduction

Within and beyond the healthcare system, people who use drugs have long been subjected to stigmatizing language, which along with prejudice, discrimination, and lack of provider education and/or training contributes to patient harm, missed opportunities for treatment, and disengagement from medical care among a population of people at increased risk of health problems [1–3]. Substance use, especially injection drug use, is one of the most highly stigmatized conditions worldwide. Those with the most serious substance use disorders are often those most affected by multiple syndemics such as personal trauma, familial or historical trauma, racism, homelessness, and mental health problems—which combine to increase vulnerability to stigma and the consequences of it [4].

Only one in ten patients with a substance use disorder has been offered treatment. Hospitalized patients who elect to leave the hospital before completing recommended treatment cite stigma and discrimination among their reasons for doing so [3]. Substance use is often cited as a contraindication to elective surgery; in our experience, it is common for such statements in the medical record to lack detail, specificity, or rationale for why the substance use (or prior use) would impact surgical candidacy. Stigma associated with substance use also occurs at a structural level and contributes to regulations and policies that limit care to people who use drugs [4]. For example, discriminatory and nonevidence-based abstinence requirements were incorporated into Medicaid coverage guidelines for direct-acting antiviral medications, limiting access to curative hepatitis C treatment among people who use drugs [5].

R. Berg (✉) · J. James · J. W. Klein
Division of General Internal Medicine, Department of Medicine, University of Washington, Seattle, WA, USA
e-mail: russberg@uw.edu; jorose@uw.edu; jaredwk@uw.edu

© The Author(s), under exclusive license to Springer Nature Switzerland AG 2023
C. J. Wong, S. L. Jackson (eds.), *The Patient-Centered Approach to Medical Note-Writing*, https://doi.org/10.1007/978-3-031-43633-8_10

As access to electronic health records expands for providers and patients alike, it is important to utilize best practices when documenting substance use. As with other conditions, inaccurate diagnoses and terms are easily propagated or simply left unchanged for years in patients' charts. Accurate, specific, respectful, and person-centered language in the electronic health record is medically appropriate and is an important step toward addressing stigmatizing beliefs and practices toward patients who use drugs. As patients who use drugs more readily access their medical records, use of medically accurate and patient-centered language about substance use may help reduce self-stigma, improve trust between patients and their providers, and increase access to needed treatment.

10.2 Substance Use: Patient-Centered Language

Research demonstrates that stigmatizing language regarding substance use may negatively influence the care provided by health professionals [2, 6]. In one study of mental health clinicians who were presented with one of two otherwise equal patient vignettes, those who read a version with *substance abuser* were more likely to blame the patient and recommend punitive measures, compared to those who read a version with the term *substance use disorder* [2]. A primary consideration in written as well as spoken language about people who use drugs is to center the person, rather than the condition, a practice referred to as "person-first" language. Patient-centered language incorporates this principle and additionally prioritizes less stigmatizing over more stigmatizing terms; patient-centered communication must also come from a spirit of respect, empathy, and collaboration.

Some terminology is embedded in the fabric of society and pervasive in casual conversations and media, making it particularly challenging to change deep-seated habits [7]. An important consideration is that substance use patterns and language continually evolve. While medical professionals should strive to use current and neutral language, it is likely that we all will fall short at times. It is best to have humility, allow grace for ourselves and others, and work to promote a professional culture that facilitates open and nonjudgmental discussion about stigma and language.

Stigmatizing language that is not specific to substance use may nevertheless have more impact on patients with substance use disorders, with additional effects due to racial biases. One study found that stigmatizing language in patients with substance use disorders was more prevalent in the notes of non-Hispanic Black patients compared to those of non-Hispanic White patients (race and ethnicity terms and data in this study were defined from EHR data) (Chap. 3) [8].

Guiding principles when documenting substance use are shown in Table 10.1. Examples of stigmatizing versus more patient-centered language are summarized in Table 10.2 and discussed below.

Table 10.1 Guiding principles when documenting substance use

• Stigma is pervasive and particularly damaging to patient-clinician relationships when substance use issues are involved
• Using person-first language is crucial to ensuring the centrality of individuals with substance use disorders
• Medically accurate language normalizes mental health and substance use issues while maintaining a neutral stance

10.2.1 Labeling

Labeling a patient as their condition can be stigmatizing (see also Chap. 3). This is particularly true for patients with substance use disorders. For example, describing a patient as a *user, addict, IVDU, drinker,* or *smoker* has the effect of equating the person with their illness. In particular, the word *user* may also convey volition or imply blame for the disorder or its complications. Some labels such as *junkie* are clearly disparaging and have no medical use—they should simply not be used. Instead, patient-centered language is preferable, e.g., *person with substance use disorder.*

Patients with substance use disorders tend to have their substance use history, even if not current, called out more than necessary. For example, it may appear in the "one-liner" at the beginning of a medical note, or at the start of the History of Present Illness, or in a summative statement that opens the Assessment and Plan (*...patient with polysubstance abuse presenting with...*) (Chaps. 7 and 13). While substance use may be important to the patient's current presentation, when not relevant its inclusion may be stigmatizing—especially if it appears to be mentioned seemingly at every opportunity or is mentioned in the absence of meaningful context.

It is important to recognize that individuals with substance use disorders are not subject to the same recommendations around language as medical professionals. For example, the terms *addict* and *alcoholic* should not be used professionally, but some patients may identify with these terms as part of their recovery process. Other terms may evolve as patients or advocacy groups work to reclaim terminology that may have been previously damaging. At the same time, clinicians may consider exploring patients' use of stigmatizing terminology, as this may represent ingrained self-stigmatization that contributes to guilt and shame, inhibiting recovery-oriented activities.

10.2.2 Up-to-Date Terminology

Use of drugs or alcohol does not necessarily mean that a person has a substance use disorder. Substance use occurs on a spectrum, as do its associated harms [9]. Substance use disorder occurs in those with chronic use leading to clinically

Table 10.2 Substance use and substance use disorder language [10, 11]

Potentially stigmatizing or outdated term(s)	More patient-centered language alternative(s)	Rationale
Labeling		
• Addict • User • IVDUer (IV drug user) • IDU (injection drug user) • IVDA (IV drug abuser) • Alcoholic	• Person with substance use disorder • Person with alcohol use disorder	Center the individual over the disease
Reformed addict	• Person who previously used [substance]	Conveys absolution rather than behavior change
Former addict	• In recovery • Long-term recovery	Better describes the process and spectrum of recovery
Non-up-to-date terminology		
• Substance abuse • Substance dependence	• Substance use disorder	Use current, medically accurate terminology (*DSM-V* rather than *DSM-IV*)
Abuse	For illicit drugs [10] • Use For prescription medications [10] • Misuse • Used other than prescribed • Use for nonmedical effects	• *Abuse* is associated with negative judgments and punishment [10]
• Clean	*For urine screen results* [10]	• *Clean* is not a clinically accurate term and has punitive connotations, in addition to pairing with its opposite, *dirty*
• Clean and sober	• Testing negative *For non-toxicology purposes* [10] • Being in remission or recovery • Abstinent from drugs • Not drinking or taking drugs • Not currently or actively using drugs	• As with terms such as *addict*, even if patients use terms such as *clean and sober*, clinicians can role model non-stigmatizing language

(continued)

Table 10.2 (continued)

Potentially stigmatizing or outdated term(s)	More patient-centered language alternative(s)	Rationale
• Opioid substitution replacement therapy • Medication-assisted treatment (MAT)	• Opioid agonist therapy • Pharmacotherapy • Addiction medication • Medication for a substance use disorder • Medication for opioid use disorder (MOUD)	May imply MOUD as a "crutch" or "trading one addiction for another" [10]
Language of policing		
Denies	• Does not use • No [substance]	Denies can be meant neutrally to a provider writing a note, but with substance use in particular, it appears accusatory
Clean/dirty urine	• Substance present/absent	Neutral language rather than stigmatizing language
Recidivism	• Return to use	Avoids implying criminality
Language of failure		
Relapse	• Return to use • Brief/temporary return to use	Relapse can imply patients are "back to square one" rather than on the path to recovery
Treatment failure	• Treatment attempt	Recognize that even seemingly unsuccessful attempts may have offered important lessons and provided individuals with significant health benefits

significant impairment or distress and is a clinical diagnosis based on 11 criteria outlined in the *Diagnostic and Statistical Manual of Mental Disorders* (*DSM*). *DSM-V* updated its terminology related to substance use disorders, replacing *substance abuse* and *substance dependence* with *substance use disorder*, which is further characterized by severity (mild, moderate, or severe). Moderate or severe substance use disorders are often referred to as *addiction*. A useful tool for recognizing addiction/substance use disorder is the "4 C's": loss of control, compulsive use, cravings, and continued use despite harm. In the absence of certainty about the diagnosis, it is recommended to use neutral language and avoid committing to a diagnosis without a rationale for doing so.

Similarly, inappropriate and potentially harmful use of drugs, prescription or otherwise, is not always "abuse." Overusing a medication for its intended purpose would best be termed "misuse," while use specifically for psychotropic effects is "abuse" [12]. It is important to understand the specific context for inappropriate substance and medication use. For example, while as-needed use of a pain medication in the evening may be appropriate use, combining it with alcohol to accentuate the psychotropic effect would be concerning. Such clarification may also illuminate next treatment steps (e.g., alternate pain treatments versus diagnosis and treatment of a substance use disorder for those meeting criteria).

10.2.3   Language of Failure

Substance use disorders in particular are subject to language that centers around failure. For example, the word *relapse* can suggest inevitability, and patients who return to substance use despite treatment are often called *treatment failures*. It is important to recognize that substance use disorders share the progressing-remitting pattern of many other chronic medical conditions. While it is natural as a provider to celebrate our patients' successes, it is easy to unintentionally create a situation in which our expectations burden patients and make it harder for them to tell us when they experience recurrent or increasing substance use.

In our written as well as spoken comments, it is helpful to use supportive but neutral terms, reinforce patients' expressed goals and motivations, and leave ourselves out of what we communicate. For sake of illustration, an extreme example is, "Doing great! I'm so proud of them. Has not used heroin in 3 months." Instead, we could simply write, "Has not used heroin in three months—goals are to remain in treatment, work toward reconnecting with daughter." It is critical that we affirm support for our patients with substance use disorders regardless of where they are in their use or recovery.

10.2.4   Language of Policing

It is not coincidental that the language of policing has crept into medical culture when speaking and writing about people who use drugs, given the long history of criminalization of substance use. For example, patients with substance use disorders may appropriately receive substance testing, but urine tests are often referred to in stigmatizing terms such as *clean* or *dirty* urine samples or *tox screens*. The term *recidivism*, typically used to refer to criminal behavior, is sometimes used to describe a return to substance use, whether illegal or not. *Denies* can suggest being accused of something and/or suggest that the patient's response is not taken at face value (see Chaps. 3 and 7). *Illicit* and *illegal* carry negative stigma, but substance use can be illegal or legal, and legality varies by state in the US (e.g., for cannabis). Further, potential harm from a given substance does not necessarily correspond with that substance's legal status.

Many people who use drugs have been incarcerated or had other interactions with the carceral system. It is important that medical providers support patients' humanity, treat substance use disorders as medical conditions, and refrain from language that conflates all substance use with criminal behavior.

10.2.5 Specificity

While labels are often too readily applied to people who use drugs, it is also common for substance use histories and associated documentation to lack substance and detail. Asking and documenting specifics about substance use is important because specifics matter—which substances, what quantity and frequency, which mode of delivery, and which harm reduction strategies. Blanket statements such as *denies illicits, no recreationals,* or *drug use: none* lack specificity and cast all substance use in the same category. More useful is documentation that includes details: e.g., ____ *does not use methamphetamines. He smokes "blues" (fentanyl pills) one to three times per day, on most days. He does not smoke cigarettes or drink alcohol.* Similarly, for alcohol use, it is best to avoid undefined terms such as *moderate drinker* or *social drinker* but instead quantify the amount. Standard drinks are defined as 12 ounces of beer, 5 ounces of wine, or 1.5 ounces of liquor.

Eliciting and documenting treatment-related details are also important. Engaging patients around specifics of treatment is important for shared decision-making and can, in the spirit of motivational interviewing, affirm self-efficacy; it can also be helpful to demonstrate patients' efforts and achievements to other members of the care team. Rather than writing that a patient is *on methadone, in treatment,* or *went to detox,* it is better to obtain and document the details of a patient's treatment. For example: ... *patient is at [name of treatment center] and receives ____ mg of methadone daily with carries on the weekend...* or ... *is in in the intensive outpatient program at [name of treatment center], attending daily from 8 am to 5 pm, attending both group sessions and individual counseling. Current medications are...*

10.3 Data Collection and Location of Substance Use History in the Chart

There is no consensus location for where a patient's substance use history should be located in an EHR or in a chart note. Within a medical note, it may be located within Social History (see Chap. 9), or as its own category, such as "Substance Use." Some EHRs have a separate window or tab in which substance use can be documented (and if desired, imported into a note). If documented in a separate part of the EHR, it is often accessible to the patient and should also use patient-first language and be updated regularly.

Substance use may further be found in the Problem List and Assessment and Plan, in which case providers should take care to use non-stigmatizing language (e.g., *tobacco use* rather than *tobacco abuse*). Whether to add substance use at all to a patient's problem list is a matter of clinical judgment. If the person has a substance use disorder, it is usually appropriate to include on the Problem List and to include in the Assessment and Plan—it is important to recognize a substance use disorder as a medical problem, anticipate associated risks or medical problems (e.g., candidacy for lung cancer screening in the setting of tobacco use), discuss harm reduction, and offer evaluation and treatment.

Data collection about substance use can be performed by both direct interview and patient surveys (either on paper or electronic). A patient who does not answer a question about substance use should not be assumed to be using that substance.

10.4 Substance Use Documentation: Additional Considerations

10.4.1 Shared Decision-Making

Shared decision-making, while part of the day-to-day work of healthcare professionals, is an especially critical skill in working with people who use drugs. As described previously, people who use drugs have faced discrimination in the healthcare system and beyond—and people with substance use disorders are not consistently offered a range of available treatments. While historically abstinence was considered the goal when it came to most substance use, alternative goals include avoiding overdose and other dangers, feeling "normal," reducing use, reducing medical or other complications of use, engaging in treatment, connecting with resources (e.g., housing, food), gaining employment, rebuilding fractured relationships, etc.—goals as varied as people are. Using motivational interviewing techniques in discussions around substance use increases trust and facilitates partnership around treatment planning. Documentation in the health record should similarly honor the motivational interviewing spirit and avoid top-down, paternalistic, or judgmental language. Reminding patients and other providers who read the chart that patients' goals, priorities, and choices are paramount can counter stigma.

Shared decision-making applies to decisions to forego, defer, or stop receiving specific treatments, as well as to decisions to engage in treatment. A common example is when patients decide to leave the hospital prior to provider-recommended discharge. *AMA discharge* or *discharge against medical advice* implies judgment and centers the providers' rather than the patients' perspective; it is preferable to simply say *discharge*, but more important is to frame such decisions with respect for patient goals and autonomy. For example, *Earlier today, patient was complaining of inadequate care and being unsatisfied…and threatening to leave AMA* portrays the patient negatively and leaves the reader with a different impression from *We were unable to adequately control ___'s pain related to their extensive open wounds, and they elected to discharge and complete a course of oral antibiotics.*

10.4.2 Substance Use and Candidacy for Surgical or Other Treatment

People with substance use and use disorders are at increased risk of physical trauma and numerous acute and chronic medical problems. Among other examples, intoxication from alcohol and/or other substances contributes to motor vehicle accidents; impairment makes people more vulnerable to assault and/or altercations; injection drug use increases risk of skin and soft tissue infections; recurrent injuries may lead to advanced arthritis; and chronic opioid use contributes to osteoporosis and hospitalization. As a result, it is common for people who use drugs to seek "elective" joint replacement for debilitating arthritis or to require post-hospital rehabilitation care.

Yet, as described previously, people with substance use disorders are subject to layers of discrimination in healthcare, and this commonly complicates candidacy for treatment (surgery, home health therapies, skilled nursing facility placement). While there may be legitimate concerns on providers' parts (e.g., ability to heal in the setting of tobacco use), there has also been normalization of discrimination against people who use drugs. Arbitrary lines are sometimes drawn, rather than carefully weighing risks, benefits, and alternatives as we offer for other conditions.

When documenting how substance use might affect patients' candidacy for placement or treatment, it is important to avoid implied acceptance or justification for discriminatory practices. If a patient's tobacco or methamphetamine use is assessed to interfere with candidacy for surgery, it is important to explain why—and to engage the patient in an honest, open, nonjudgmental discussion around substance use and goals. Chart notes that simply state *still smoking, not a candidate for hip surgery* may be perceived to slam the door on a patient, potentially dashing longstanding hopes.

10.4.3 Buprenorphine and Methadone for Opioid Use Disorder

It is common for providers to misunderstand why a patient takes buprenorphine or methadone, which can be used for both pain and opioid use disorder. If a patient takes one of these medications for opioid use disorder, it should be recognized that they are taking a life-saving medication and that the decision to taper or stop it is a serious one that should be made using shared decision-making involving qualified providers. At times, providers without training in addiction medicine will make—and document—ill-advised recommendations to taper or stop an opioid, without understanding what the medication is for and what the consequences of that messaging may be. Even if patients do not follow such advice, such messages may undermine the patient's trust in healthcare and/or reinforce stigma.

10.5   Conclusion

Substance use and substance use disorders are some of the most stigmatized conditions in healthcare. There are language practices that are common to other recommendations in this book, but also important considerations specific to, or more often applied to, patients with substance use disorders, as reviewed in this chapter. While updating documentation practices cannot by itself optimize the health of patients with these conditions, patient-centered language is one important aspect of care that can be synergistic with our treatment for patients with substance use and substance use disorders.

References

1. van Boekel LC, Brouwers EP, van Weeghel J, Garretsen HF. Stigma among health professionals towards patients with substance use disorders and its consequences for healthcare delivery: systematic review. Drug Alcohol Depend. 2013;131(1–2):23–35. https://doi.org/10.1016/j.drugalcdep.2013.02.018.
2. Kelly JF, Westerhoff CM. Does it matter how we refer to individuals with substance-related conditions? A randomized study of two commonly used terms. Int J Drug Policy. 2010;21(3):202–7. https://doi.org/10.1016/j.drugpo.2009.10.010.
3. Simon R, Snow R, Wakeman S. Understanding why patients with substance use disorders leave the hospital against medical advice: a qualitative study. Subst Abus. 2020;41(4):519–25. https://doi.org/10.1080/08897077.2019.1671942.
4. Committee on the Science of Changing Behavioral Health Social Norms; Board on Behavioral, Cognitive, and Sensory Sciences; Division of Behavioral and Social Sciences and Education; National Academies of Sciences, Engineering, and Medicine. Ending discrimination against people with mental and substance use disorders: the evidence for stigma change. Washington, DC: National Academies Press (US); 2016. https://doi.org/10.17226/23442.
5. Liao JM, Fischer MA. Restrictions of hepatitis C treatment for substance-using Medicaid patients: cost versus ethics. Am J Public Health. 2017;107(6):893–9. https://doi.org/10.2105/AJPH.2017.303748.
6. Ashford RD, Brown AM, McDaniel J, Curtis B. Biased labels: an experimental study of language and stigma among individuals in recovery and health professionals. Subst Use Misuse. 2019;54(8):1376–84. https://doi.org/10.1080/10826084.2019.1581221.
7. Atayde AMP, Hauc SC, Bessette LG, Danckers H, Saitz R. Changing the narrative: a call to end stigmatizing terminology related to substance use disorders. Addict Res Theory. 2021;29(5):359–62. https://doi.org/10.1080/16066359.2021.1875215.
8. Himmelstein G, Bates D, Zhou L. Examination of stigmatizing language in the electronic health record. JAMA Netw Open. 2022;5(1):e2144967. https://doi.org/10.1001/jamanetworkopen.2021.44967.
9. American Psychiatric Association: Diagnostic and Statistical Manual of Mental Disorders, Fifth Edition, Text Revision. Washington, DC, American Psychiatric Association, 2022.
10. National Institute on Drug Abuse. Words matter—terms to use and avoid when talking about addiction. https://nida.nih.gov/nidamed-medical-health-professionals/health-professions-education/words-matter-terms-to-use-avoid-when-talking-about-addiction#ref. Accessed 19 May 2023.

11. Ashford RD, Brown AM, Curtis B. Substance use, recovery, and linguistics: the impact of word choice on explicit and implicit bias. Drug Alcohol Depend. 2018;189:131–8. https://doi. org/10.1016/j.drugalcdep.2018.05.005.
12. Smith SM, Dart RC, Katz NP, Paillard F, Adams EH, Comer SD, Degroot A, Edwards RR, Haddox DJ, Jaffe JH, Jones CM, Kleber HD, Kopecky EA, Markman JD, Montoya ID, O'Brien C, Roland CL, Stanton M, Strain EC, Vorsanger G, Wasan AD, Weiss RD, Turk DC, Dworkin RH. Classification and definition of misuse, abuse, and related events in clinical trials: ACTTION systematic review and recommendations. Pain. 2013;154(11):2287–96. https:// doi.org/10.1016/j.pain.2013.05.053.

Chapter 11
Mental Health

Russell Berg, Jocelyn James, and Jared W. Klein

11.1 Introduction

Clinicians may experience uncertainty or discomfort when documenting about mental health in the era of Open Notes and the 21st Century Cures Act mandating greater access to medical notes [1]. Without diagnostic procedures to confirm psychiatric disorders, our assessments in this realm may seem more subjective—a significant concern given the potential stigma and other negative consequences that a mental health diagnosis can invoke. Evidence from inpatient consultations to psychiatry suggests that nonpsychiatrists are just as likely to misdiagnose psychiatric disorders as to get the diagnosis correct [2]. Even descriptors of psychiatric symptoms or behaviors can be inaccurate and subject to the influence of stigma and bias. Stigmatizing language in clinical documentation leads to less trusting patient-provider relationships, more difficult therapeutic alliances, and the potential for worse outcomes for patients [3].

At the same time, when notes are respectful and match the content of clinical encounters, this can engender greater trust between patients and clinicians [4]. There is evidence that primary care patients with access to their notes have improved understanding of their health and engagement in care, whether or not they have a mental health diagnosis [5]. Principles of documentation for encounters focused on mental health are shared with all medical fields—use patient-centered, specific language and use patient quotations only when doing so provides important information and enhances the voice of the patient. It is possible as providers to leverage our notes to build trust and strengthen therapeutic relationships with those who have mental illness.

R. Berg (✉) · J. James · J. W. Klein
Division of General Internal Medicine, Department of Medicine, University of Washington, Seattle, WA, USA
e-mail: russberg@uw.edu; jorose@uw.edu; jaredwk@uw.edu

© The Author(s), under exclusive license to Springer Nature Switzerland AG 2023

C. J. Wong, S. L. Jackson (eds.), *The Patient-Centered Approach to Medical Note-Writing*, https://doi.org/10.1007/978-3-031-43633-8_11

147

11.2   Terminology

Behavioral health is considered an umbrella term that encompasses both mental health (diagnoses such as depression and anxiety) and a variety of other health domains such as substance use (discussed in Chap. 10), exercise, sexual history, social interactions, and diet, although there is no consensus definition as to what components are included. Many people use the terms *mental health* and *behavioral health* interchangeably in common speech. While "mental" is derived from the Latin "mens" (mind), describing awareness and an internal experience or feeling, "behavior" implies an external observer of one's conduct. It is our position to prefer the term "mental health" when concerning psychiatric conditions.

11.3   Use Patient-Centered Rather Than
Disease-Centered Terms

Choosing patient-centered rather than disease-centered language gives primacy to the person rather than to their condition. This is especially important in the context of mental health, given the historical mistreatment and isolation of those with mental illness [6]. Mental health conditions in particular tend to become affixed to the patient carrying those conditions—these labels can occur either as a unique word (*schizophrenic*) or as a word tied closely with the person (*bipolar patient*) (Table 11.1, see also Chaps. 3 and 7).

11.4   Mental Health in the History of Present Illness (HPI)

The narrative history for mental health conditions should have similar attention to patient-centered, nonstigmatizing language as discussed in Chap. 7. Note however that the use of quotations may be different: a psychiatric history as performed by psychiatrists has a tradition of using frequent quotations in an effort to capture the patient's voice. When used in that sense, quotations do not necessarily convey doubt, disapproval, or condescension, as they may in other contexts (Chaps. 3 and 7). However, a substantial portion of mental health care is provided by clinicians who are not formally trained as psychiatrists or psychologists. For providers without such advanced training in psychiatry, when documenting mental health in the HPI, they should be careful to double check their use of quotations to ensure that the purpose is to enhance the patient's history rather than question it.

Table 11.1 Avoiding the use of labels in patients with mental health disorders [7]

Potentially stigmatizing or labeling term	Alternative	Rationale
… 30-year-old bipolar patient with hypertension and frequent UTIs presenting today …	… 30-year-old patient with hypertension, bipolar disorder, and frequent UTIs presenting today …	By placing *bipolar* before the word *patient*, it effectively labels the patient and assigns more importance to this diagnosis. Instead, include (if relevant) among the other health conditions
… is a 40-year-old schizophrenic presenting with …	… is a 40-year-old person with schizophrenia presenting with …	*Schizophrenic* is a label, similar to *diabetic*
… psych patient …	… patient with [diagnosis] …	This is more commonly spoken than written (see Chap. 16 for discussion of Oral Case Presentations). Referring to a patient as a *psych patient* reduces their personhood and creates a stereotyped impression
… is a borderline patient who …	… is a patient with a history of borderline personality disorder who …	Similar to *bipolar patient* above. Note also that in some cases, a patient is labeled as borderline because of certain behaviors but does not actually carry a confirmed diagnosis of borderline personality disorder

Some of the examples above are adapted from Jensen et al. [7]

11.5 Mental Health in the Exam Portion of the Note

The mental status exam is known as the physical exam for psychiatrists—for those formally trained in psychiatry, the mental status exam is a rigorous synthesis of observations. Those who do not have advanced training in psychiatry or psychology may unintentionally use historically stigmatizing or imprecise terms when documenting a mental health exam.

Documenting general appearance and behavior may be most problematic for those without psychiatry training. Assessments of appearance and grooming, which are often subject to cultural norms, may be mentioned without serving a clear purpose. If a formal mental status exam is indicated, it is better to integrate observations about general appearance or behavior into this section rather than placing them under "General" in the first part of the physical exam. Otherwise, it is usually more appropriate to refrain from commenting on grooming (see Chap. 12).

Some behavioral descriptors (e.g., guardedness, hostility, and agitation) may convey negative implications to readers—patients and other providers alike. It is important to include such terms only when trained to apply them appropriately within the context of a psychiatric assessment. Inaccurate, biased, or simply unnecessary use of such terms can be harmful, especially if used in the absence of a thorough mental status exam.

A "Psychiatric" or "Psych" section of the physical exam may prompt providers to include off-handed or vague descriptors; those without psychiatric training should be careful to avoid entering terms with meaning they may not fully understand or intend. It is likely that for many note templates, a Psychiatric section was included in the Physical Exam even when a patient is seen for non-mental-health-related concerns because of billing and coding incentives, increasing the risk for inappropriate psychiatric "exam" documentation. Fortunately, these requirements have eased and providers should feel empowered to not document a psychiatric exam if a thorough mental status exam was neither indicated nor performed (see Chap. 12).

It is also important to be attuned to our own implicit biases, to cultural differences, and to the many ways that experiences of racism affect our patients' behavior. A study of inpatient admission notes found that stigmatizing language appeared more often in admission notes of Black patients, in comparison to those of White patients (race was defined by EHR data) [8]. Animated ways of speaking may be misinterpreted as *agitation*; patients who have ample reasons to mistrust medical providers may be labeled as *guarded*; patients who are not stereotypically expressive in the medical exam room (an uncomfortable setting for many patients) may be inappropriately pathologized as having a *flat affect*.

While documentation of mental-health-related descriptors in the physical exam can be harmful when inaccurate, vague, or irrelevant (Table 11.2), a properly conducted mental status exam is fundamental to a comprehensive psychiatric assessment. Approaches to a mental status exam vary, but some commonly included elements are appearance and behavior, eye contact, motor activity, mood, affect,

Table 11.2 Imprecise or stigmatizing language pertaining to mental health in the exam portion of the note

Potentially stigmatizing language	Alternative	Rationale
General: unkempt, no acute distress	General: no acute distress	People can have a wide range of appearance—unkempt or disheveled to one person may be normal to another. If grooming is deemed important, consider documenting formally as part of the mental status exam
General: disheveled, lying in gurney, no acute distress	General: lying in gurney, no acute distress	
General: agitated, anxious	General: no acute distress	Agitated and anxious are not specific. They do not describe what the patient is doing to merit the description of being agitated. If important to document as an exam finding, it is usually better to describe in a mental status exam
Psych: normal affect	[Leave out]	If a patient is seen for reasons not related to mental health, it is likely not necessary to document their affect at all
Psych: tangential, not pressured	[Leave out]	Some patients are simply not practiced at telling their history in the way that is easiest for medical professionals to understand (avoid the term *poor historian*, as the clinician is the "historian", not the patient). If their history is so tangential to merit a mental status exam, it is better to do a formal mental status exam rather than mention it in this manner

speech, thought process and content, current suicidality (ideas, plan, intent), cognition, insight, and judgment [9].

11.6   Potential Harm to a Patient from Reading Their Note

Some have concern that access to Open Notes for mental health documentation may weaken the therapeutic relationship. A qualitative study of Veterans found that reading clinical notes can either weaken or strengthen trust in a mental health provider, and that factors associated with improved trust included accuracy of documentation and transparency (e.g., absence of surprise psychiatric diagnoses) [4].

Some experts have also expressed concern that persons with "delusional symptoms and other common diagnoses such as bipolar, schizophrenia, active suicidal ideation, personality disorders… may be destabilized if (they) had access to medical notes" [10]. Federal law regulating patient access to medical records allows for withholding of information if it will prevent harm by doing so; however, the withholding of HIPAA protected EHI must be limited, justified, and substantially reduce risk of harm [11]. Many EHRs will prompt a note writer to document why a note is not to be shared with a patient. While there are limited data on overall "information blocking" on a systems level [12], and some data on formal patient complaints [13], it is unknown whether patients with psychiatric conditions have their notes hidden more often that patients with other conditions.

Note that psychotherapy notes are an exception to the "information blocking" Cures Act Rule, as they are considered personal notes of the therapist; they are not required to be viewable by the patient, and are also not shared with other providers without patient authorization.

11.7   Conclusion

Patients with mental health conditions often already experience stigma in society and health-care settings. Documentation practices that avoid labeling patients as their disease are especially important for patients with psychiatric disorders. As a substantial amount of mental health assessment and treatment is conducted by providers who are not psychiatrists, it is critical that training include patient-centered documentation techniques for the patient history and exam, including being judicious about when to include the psychiatric exam. Providers also need to be aware that government regulations in the United States allow for notes not to be shared with patients if there is substantial risk of harm. With implementation of the recommendations outlined in this chapter, it is hoped that the documentation of mental health will be more patient-centered and provide an improved healing environment for our patients.

References

1. The 21st Century Cures Act. https://www.congress.gov/114/plaws/publ255/PLAW-114publ255.pdf. Accessed 27 May 2023.
2. AlSalem M, AlHarbi MA, Badeghiesh A, Tourian L. Accuracy of initial psychiatric diagnoses given by nonpsychiatric physicians: a retrospective chart review. Medicine (Baltimore). 2020;99(51):e23708. https://doi.org/10.1097/MD.0000000000023708.
3. Dobscha SK, Denneson LM, Jacobson LE, Williams HB, Cromer R, Woods S. VA mental health clinician experiences and attitudes toward OpenNotes. Gen Hosp Psychiatry. 2016;38:89–93.
4. Cromer R, Denneson LM, Pisciotta M, Williams H, Woods S, Dobscha SK. Trust in mental health clinicians among patients who access clinical notes online. Psychiatr Serv. 2017;68(5):520–3.
5. Klein J, Peacock S, Tsui JI, O'Neill SF, DesRoches CM, Elmore JG. Perceptions of primary care notes by patients with mental health diagnoses. Ann Fam Med. 2018;16(4):343–5.
6. Shattell MM. Stigmatizing language with unintended meanings: "persons with mental illness" or "mentally ill persons"? Issues Ment Health Nurs. 2009;30(3):199. https://doi.org/10.1080/01612840802694668.
7. Jensen ME, Pease EA, Lambert K, Hickman DR, Robinson O, McCoy KT, Barut JK, Musker KM, Olive D, Noll C, Ramirez J, Cogliser D, King JK. Championing person-first language: a call to psychiatric mental health nurses. J Am Psychiatr Nurses Assoc. 2013;19(3):146–51. https://doi.org/10.1177/1078390313489729.
8. Himmelstein G, Bates D, Zhou L. Examination of stigmatizing language in the electronic health record. JAMA Netw Open. 2022;5(1):e2144967. https://doi.org/10.1001/jamanetworkopen.2021.44967.
9. Silverman JJ, Galanter M, Jackson-Triche M, Jacobs DG, Lomax JW II, Riba MB, et al. The APA practice guidelines for the psychiatric evaluation of adults. 3rd ed. Arlington, VA: American Psychiatric Association; 2016. ISBN 978-0-89042-465-0. https://psychiatryonline.org/doi/epdf/10.1176/appi.books.9780890426760. Accessed 25 Feb 2023.
10. Blease C, Torous J, Kharko A, DesRoches CM, Harcourt K, O'Neill S, Salmi L, Wachenheim D, Hägglund M. Preparing patients and clinicians for open notes in mental health: qualitative inquiry of international experts. JMIR Ment Health. 2021;8(4):e27397. https://doi.org/10.2196/27397.
11. The Office of the National Coordinator for Health Information Technology. Cures act final rule: information blocking exceptions. https://www.healthit.gov/sites/default/files/2022-07/InformationBlockingExceptions.pdf. Accessed 20 May 2023.
12. Everson J, Patel V, Adler-Milstein J. Information blocking remains prevalent at the start of 21st Century Cures Act: results from a survey of health information exchange organizations. J Am Med Inform Assoc. 2021;28(4):727–32. https://doi.org/10.1093/jamia/ocaa323.
13. HealthIT.gov. Information blocking claims: by the numbers. https://www.healthit.gov/data/quickstats/information-blocking-claims-numbers. Accessed 20 May 2023.

Chapter 12
The Review of Systems and the Physical Exam

Scott Hagan and Anna F. Hagan

12.1 The Review of Systems

The purpose of the Review of Systems (ROS) section of clinical notes is to assess comprehensively for new symptoms that may not have been discovered during the initial history taking. In training programs, health-care practitioners learn the complete ROS using a series of questions in broad categories such as constitutional (fevers, chills, fatigue), skin (rash), pulmonary (cough, wheezing), cardiovascular (chest pain, palpitations), gastrointestinal (nausea, diarrhea), et cetera [1]. Through a structured approach to symptom review, additional symptoms may lead the clinician to consider alternative diagnoses.

12.1.1 Clinical Use Versus Coding/Billing Guidelines

While the educational value of a complete ROS is clear, the benefit in clinical practice of pursuing and documenting a detailed ROS in many situations is uncertain [2]. Pertinent positives and negatives should be discussed within the History of Present Illness (HPI), often without the clinical need to have a separate category for ROS. The ROS may be more useful when taking a full history and physical with a new outpatient, a newly admitted inpatient, or when assessing a challenging diagnostic case.

S. Hagan (✉) · A. F. Hagan
Division of General Internal Medicine, Department of Medicine, University of Washington, Seattle, WA, USA
e-mail: scotthag@uw.edu; annafahy@uw.edu

© The Author(s), under exclusive license to Springer Nature Switzerland AG 2023
C. J. Wong, S. L. Jackson (eds.), *The Patient-Centered Approach to Medical Note-Writing*, https://doi.org/10.1007/978-3-031-43633-8_12

   In the United States, providers have historically been required to document a ROS as a discrete section of the note because of Center for Medicare and Medicaid Services (CMS) documentation guidelines dating back to the 1990s [3]. These guidelines delineated the following 14 categories: Constitutional; Eyes; Ears, Nose, Mouth, Throat; Cardiovascular; Respiratory; Gastrointestinal; Genitourinary; Musculoskeletal; Integumentary; Neurologic; Psychiatric; Endocrine; Hematologic/ Lymphatic; Allergic/Immunologic. However, these systems categories are not necessarily intuitive or precisely defined. For example, breast symptoms are intended to be part of the "integumentary" system although most providers likely consider breast symptoms anatomically; sweats could be a symptom of many systems, including constitutional, endocrine, or hematologic; exertional symptoms could be due to cardiovascular, respiratory, or even hematologic etiologies such as anemia.

   Nevertheless, these categories became enshrined at least in part because of coding requirements, resulting in excessive documentation that is often either fraudulent or misleading. Because the number of ROS categories addressed and documented was incorporated as one element to determine the level of billing, providers were incentivized to include more ROS in their notes, often resulting in an unnecessary level of symptom review for the clinical situation. Combining this incentive with the widespread use of standardized note templates with a comprehensive ROS, fraudulent documentation of a thorough ROS is common. Indeed, one study found that only 39% of documented ROS findings were confirmed by observational data [4]. Further, CMS did not define the minimum amount of symptom review in each ROS category to count that category toward the minimum ROS for different billing levels. There are potentially dozens of questions in different ROS categories that could be reviewed [1]; therefore, the statement "all other systems negative" lacks precision and could be misinterpreted as a much broader symptom review than was conducted in the visit.

   With changes to evaluation and management (E/M) coding criteria in 2021 for office visits and in 2023 for inpatient visits in the United States [5, 6], documentation of an ROS section is no longer an element that determines the billing level of a clinical encounter. Electronic Health Record (EHR) note templates, patient questionnaires, and medical training may take time to implement these changes. Some authors advocate eliminating the ROS altogether because of its lack of evidence base, its diminished role in billing, and its potential detraction from time spent performing other needed clinical activities [7]. If a clinician feels that a separate ROS is clinically useful for a patient evaluation, then they should document what symptoms are asked, and not feel compelled to ask all categories as previously delineated for billing purposes. Statements such as "Complete ROS is negative except as noted in the HPI" should be avoided, for the reasons described above.

12.1.2 Patient-Centered Language in the Review of Systems

If a clinician opts to include a partial or comprehensive review of systems, they do not need to adhere strictly to the former categories that were established for billing/coding purposes. When documenting, providers may free-text or dictate the ROS, or as is common practice with many EHRs, use ROS fields with discrete choice elements. There are several common patient-centered language issues to consider when documenting an ROS. Many of these are similar to language used in the HPI, as a review of systems may be included in that section (see also Chap. 7).

Endorses/Denies A common practice in the ROS is to use the word "endorse" for positive symptoms or findings, and "denies" for those that are absent. While some patients are likely accustomed to such medical jargon, others may find the word *denies* to be disrespectful [8]. Additionally a *denial* of a symptom or behavior may be interpreted differently by context: for example, a patient may not feel disrespected at *denying* having chest pain but may feel not believed if they *deny drug use*. While the terms *endorse* and *deny* are not by themselves always problematic, they are also not actual medical terms (unlike, e.g., "orthopnea" or "fluctuance"—terms which patients may not understand but which have specific medical definitions) and therefore, other than serving as a medical style, do not serve any clinical purpose. A simpler practice would be to simply write that a patient has or does not have a particular symptom; if written in list form, then symptoms may be documented as "present" and "absent."

Quotations As discussed elsewhere in this book (see Chaps. 3 and 7), quotations should be used with care. Quotations sometimes appear in the ROS. If used, the clinician should use them with attention to context, as their selective use can appear to cast doubt on the patient's history. For example:

ROS: … Musculoskeletal: "12/10" knee pain. …

The above may give the impression that the note writer believes the patient is exaggerating their amount of pain. In some cases, quotations can serve to make the patient's narrative richer by using their own words—if used, it is recommended that the note writer read over the note critically for what impression the quotation leaves. Additionally, if a quotation is used, the note writer should also be completely certain of the accuracy of the quotation, as being misquoted can be a source of a patient's feeling disrespected [8].

12.2 The Physical Exam

The physical exam section is a key component of the objective portion of a clinical note.

12.2.1   Interaction Between Billing/Coding and Physical Exam in Medical Notes

To consider why medical notes, especially the exam portion, seem to include so many sections, it is important to review how these note writing practices developed. Similar to the ROS, medical notes may be influenced not only by what is medically useful, but also by the coding requirements of payors. The 1997 CMS guidelines defined four levels of physical examination based on the number and depth of organ systems examined and documented [9]. The history, physical exam, and medical decision making were considered the three main criteria for determining a level of service, using the highest levels of two out of the three categories. For the physical exam, there were four levels of examination: "problem focused," "expanded problem focused," "detailed," and "comprehensive." In order to qualify for a "comprehensive" examination (which was generally required for the highest level of service), either a "complete" examination of a single organ or a "general multisystem examination" of at least nine organ systems or body areas was required [9]. These organ systems were: Constitutional, Eyes, Ears/Nose/Mouth/Throat, Neck, Respiratory, Cardiovascular, Chest (Breasts), Gastrointestinal (Abdomen), Genitourinary, Lymphatic, Musculoskeletal, Skin, Neurologic, and Psychiatric. Generations of medical notes including EHR templates followed suit and adopted these categories. While these categories are generally useful, they do not always fit a clinical evaluation—for example, peripheral edema is part of Cardiovascular in this system, but there are more causes for edema than cardiovascular—rigid note systems may reinforce more limited differential diagnoses than are appropriate.

Although clinicians are only supposed to perform and document examinations that are clinically indicated, these coding categories influenced the layout and content of clinical notes. EHRs allow clinicians to import pre-populated physical examinations, or to copy/paste a physical examination from a prior note. This capability increases the likelihood that aspects of the exam that the clinician did not perform during the visit are included in the note [10]. If a patient reads a note and discovers that portions of the physical exam were documented but not performed, not only is this documentation fraudulent, but it also can lead to a breakdown of trust in the clinician-patient relationship. In one study of resident physicians comparing observation of clinical encounters to subsequent documentation, only 53% of documented physical exam findings were confirmed by concurrent observation [4]. It is of paramount importance to include only portions of the physical exam that are performed during the encounter.

12.2.2   Objective Language in the Physical Examination

The physical examination portion of the note is meant to be a descriptive review of exam findings, as opposed to an interpretation of these findings. The clinician should thus describe what they are observing using neutral language, without making diagnostic conclusions. Further, the use of medical terminology in the physical exam portion of the note is appropriate; however, it is important to be mindful of using language that could be harmful to patients, even if unintentional. When documenting a physical examination, the following questions should be considered:

- Is the exam important to document? As noted above, many templates include an extensive list of organ systems that may not be relevant to a clinical encounter. Listing an exam element that is not necessary contributes to "note bloat"—for example, a stable outpatient presenting with a musculoskeletal problem usually does not need to have exam elements that are observed incidentally such as a respiratory exam that states that the patient has *normal respiratory effort* or is *not using accessory muscles*—while factually true, such unnecessary exams do not add clinical value. Further, the custom of adding exam elements that are unnecessary risks including terms that are imprecise—for example, adding *Normal appearance* under Constitutional is not specific.
- Is the examination description objective? For example, general appearance descriptors such as "pleasant" or "dressed appropriately" are not well defined and subject to bias.
- Is the examination description neutral in language? Not only can language lack objectivity and specificity, but it can be harmful to patients. For example, calling a patient "elderly" as part of their physical examination is not specific and can give the impression that the note writer is stereotyping the patient rather than considering them as an individual.

Table 12.1 provides practical tips for common language to avoid in the physical exam, with suggestions for alternatives.

Table 12.1 Patient-centered language in the physical exam

Section (example)[a]	Subject	Words to avoid	Patient-centered language	Discussion
General	Age descriptors	• Middle-aged elderly • Appears older than stated age	[Leave out]	The age is known from elsewhere in the chart. Age descriptions are unnecessary and may result in age discrimination or the appearance of age discrimination. *Older than* or *Younger than* stated age is not objective—people have a wide range of appearances and comparison to expected norms is highly subject to biases. If *appears older than stated age* is intended to comment on a patient's ill-appearance, then objective assessment of that ill-appearance would be more useful.

(continued)

Table 12.1 (continued)

Section (example)[a]	Subject	Words to avoid	Patient-centered language	Discussion
	Gender	• Woman • Man	[Leave out]	A clinician cannot interpret an individual's gender based on the physical exam. This language is unnecessary.
	Body habitus	• Obese • Thin • Fat	[Leave out]	While "obese" does have a definition (BMI over 30), it is not necessary to put in general or constitutional, as BMI data may be found in vital signs. If important clinically, may describe body habitus in other body areas. ("temporal wasting," "pannus overlying inguinal folds")
	General appearance	• Ill-appearance • Toxic-appearing • Normal appearance • Non-toxic	• Diaphoretic • Rigors visible in the jaw and hands • Short of breath	These interpretive descriptions also lack specificity. Instead, the clinician should simply describe what they observe
	Demeanor or attitude	• Pleasant • Unpleasant • Cooperative • Uncooperative • Agitated	[Leave out]	These words describe the clinician's interpretation based on their interaction and do not add clinical relevance. Further, they raise concern for the bias the clinician may have towards the patient
	Grooming	• Well-groomed • Disheveled	[Leave out]	Grooming assessment has been recommended in some versions of the psychiatric mental status exam (see discussion below). Its role in general appearance and its clinical utility is not clear, and is subject to bias regarding perceived societal norms.

Table 12.1 (continued)

Section (example)[a]	Subject	Words to avoid	Patient-centered language	Discussion
	Race or ethnicity	• African-American, Hispanic, Asian, etc. • Skin appropriate color for ethnicity	[Leave out]	The physical exam cannot identify an individual's race or ethnicity. If a description of an individual's skin color is relevant to the clinical evaluation, it should be described in the Skin section of the exam using an objective measure such as the Fitzpatrick scale.
Head/ears/ nose/throat	Oral cavity exam	Poor dentition	Multiple caries, gingival hypertrophy, edentulous	Interpretive. If clinically relevant, consider an objective description of findings in the oropharynx.
Neurologic		Grossly non-focal	Symmetric facial gestures, speech clear, extra-ocular movements intact	*Grossly* does not add value and may be misinterpreted by the patient as unpleasant. *Non-focal* implies that a complete neurological exam was performed. Instead describe the pertinent, specific findings.
Cardiac	Limitations of an exam	Could not assess neck veins due to patient's body habitus	Neck veins were not visible.	The language implies that the patient's neck tissue is the reason that the exam is not possible, rather than other feasible explanations such as volume depletion.
Respiratory	Normality	Normal lungs	Clear bilaterally No crackles or wheezes	*Normal* in some cases may not pose any problem; however, it does not make clear what examination was conducted. Suggest documenting the relevant positive or negative findings. Similarly, using *abnormal* in an exam may be both unnecessarily negative and not useful clinically (e.g., *body habitus: abnormal*)—see Chap. 5 for further discussion.

(continued)

Table 12.1 (continued)

Section (example)[a]	Subject	Words to avoid	Patient-centered language	Discussion
Abdomen	Body habitus	Obese	[Leave out or:] Waist-to-hip ratio: __ Pannus with redness, induration, tenderness inferiorly, without fluctuance	*Obese* is an unnecessary descriptor in either general appearance or other exam areas. If clinically indicated, body habitus should be described objectively. For example, if assessing metabolic risk, central adiposity and waist circumference, or waist to hip ratio, may be helpful. If assessing for a possible skin infection, description of the location with respect to a patient's pannus may be helpful. Documenting "obese" or "thin" by itself adds little additional value to the objective data and may be stigmatizing × some patients.
	Declining an exam	Refuses pelvic/ rectal exam	Preferred not to have a rectal exam today. [Document discussion]	*Refuses* has a negative connotation. Preferred language is *declines* or *defers*, with *defer* only being used if the patient truly agreed to a potential exam at a later date. Documenting the discussion is helpful to understand the reasons for a patient not wanting to receive a part of an exam.
Psychiatric		• Anxious • Agitated • Cooperative • Uncooperative		Rather than brief descriptors, if a mental status exam is relevant, suggest conducting a systematic mental status examination per psychiatric guidelines (see below)

[a] The cardiac, respiratory, abdomen, and GI/GU examples above are to illustrate potentially problematic language and are not specific to those organ systems

12.2.3 The Mental Status Exam

A detailed discussion of the psychiatric mental status examination is beyond the scope of this book. When it comes to documenting patient characteristics that fall under the mental status exam, it is first worthwhile to consider whether it needs to be documented at all. If a patient returns for routine follow-up of a medical condition such as diabetes or hypertension, it is likely not clinically relevant to document that they had a normal affect, or appeared euthymic, or were cooperative. If mental health concerns were raised by the patient or otherwise found by the clinician (as, e.g., during the interview or via appropriate screening tools), then it is generally better to include the psychiatric exam systematically as a mental status exam.

It is also worth noting that the mental status exam has varying teachings—while some advocate for including race, gender, and grooming, the American Psychiatric Association does not include any of these descriptors in their guidelines for the general appearance section of the physical examination. Rather, race and ethnicity may be relevant as part of Social History, and grooming is not mentioned at all [11].

12.3 Use of Fonts

With the EHR, some note templating automatically adjusts fonts for positive or negative findings in the ROS or PE. While this practice can make it easier to identify pertinent positives and negatives, it may also reinforce stigmatizing language, if present.

Example: A physical exam using color fonts:

Appearance: She is **obese**. She is not ill-appearing or diaphoretic.

Example: An ROS using italics

Psychiatric: *anxious, drug use*.

Unless EHR templating uses patient-centered language principles, it is a better practice not to call out note elements with color, italic, or other font choices (see also Chap. 6).

12.4 Summary

The Review of Systems is not always clinically necessary; it no longer has a prominent role in billing and coding in the United States. When used, the ROS should include only the systems that are relevant to a clinical situation and should employ patient-centered language. The Physical Exam should include what is relevant to a clinical evaluation, and there are no longer incentives to include more exam systems than are necessary. Patient-centered language in the physical examination section of a medical note includes avoiding judgmental terms and including only objective findings. Table 12.2 includes a summary of key points for using patient-centered language in the ROS and PE.

Table 12.2 Key points for using patient-centered language in the ROS and PE

• A separate section of a medical note for the ROS is not required in most clinical situations. Pertinent positives and negatives may be incorporated into the HPI
• Avoid writing *ROS negative except as stated in HPI* as this statement is not necessary for billing purposes and lacks precision
• As with the HPI, the use of the terms *endorse* and *deny* is not necessary; *deny* may have negative connotations
• The PE no longer needs to adhere to the prior 1997 CMS guidelines, which dictated the types of systems and depth required for various billing levels
• The PE often contains subjective or poorly defined terms—best practices are to limit the PE to objective findings that are relevant to a patient's care
• EHR templates may still be based on outdated incentives for overdocumentation or lack patient-centered language

References

1. Bickley LS, Szilagyi PG, Hoffman RM. Bates's guide to physical examination and history taking. 13th ed. Philadelphia, PA: Wolters Kluwer; 2021.
2. Hendrickson MA, Melton GB, Pitt MB. The review of systems, the electronic health record, and billing. JAMA. 2019;322(2):115–6.
3. Centers for Medicare and Medicaid Services. 1995 documentation guidelines for evaluation and management services. https://www.cms.gov/outreach-and-education/medicare-learning-network-mln/mlnedwebguide/downloads/95docguidelines.pdf. Accessed 20 Feb 2023.
4. Berdahl CT, Moran GJ, McBride O, Santini AM, Verzhbinsky IA, Schriger DL. Concordance between electronic clinical documentation and physicians' observed behavior. JAMA Netw Open. 2019;2(9):e1911390.
5. American Medical Association. 2021 CPT® evaluation and management (E/M) office or other outpatient (99202–99215) and prolonged services (99354, 99355, 99356, 99417) code and guideline changes. https://www.ama-assn.org/system/files/2019-06/cpt-office-prolonged-svs-code-changes.pdf. Accessed 26 Apr 2023.
6. American Medical Association. 2023 CPT® evaluation and management (E/M) code and guideline changes. https://www.ama-assn.org/system/files/2023-e-m-descriptors-guidelines.pdf. Accessed 26 Apr 2023.
7. Barry MJ, Tseng C. Moving to more evidence-based primary care encounters: a farewell to the review of systems. JAMA. 2022;328(15):1495–6. https://doi.org/10.1001/jama.2022.18346.
8. Fernández L, Fossa A, Dong Z, et al. Words matter: what do patients find judgmental or offensive in outpatient notes? J Gen Intern Med. 2021;36(9):2571–8.
9. Centers for Medicare and Medicaid Services. 1997 documentation guidelines for evaluation and management services. https://www.cms.gov/outreach-and-education/medicare-learning-network-mln/mlnedwebguide/downloads/97docguidelines.pdf. Accessed 20 Feb 2023.
10. Bell SK, Delbanco T, Elmore JG, et al. Frequency and types of patient-reported errors in electronic health record ambulatory care notes. JAMA Netw Open. 2020;3(6):e205867.
11. Silverman JJ, Galanter M, Jackson-Triche M, Jacobs DG, Lomax JW II, Riba MB, et al. The APA practice guidelines for the psychiatric evaluation of adults. 3rd ed. Arlington, VA: American Psychological Association. https://psychiatryonline.org/doi/epdf/10.1176/appi.books.9780890426760. Accessed 25 Feb 2023.

Chapter 13
The Assessment and Plan

Margaret Isaac and Sarah Leyde

13.1 Introduction

One challenge in documentation is the multiple potential audiences whom the medical record serves. The writer, the patient, and other health professionals involved in the patient's care are the primary audience, but many others may read the patient's chart, including researchers, administrators, payers, quality improvement staff, caregivers, and even attorneys in medicolegal situations [1].

The Assessment and Plan (A/P) is arguably one of the most important parts of the medical database. It contains not just the clinician's formulation of the patient's concerns, but also the differential diagnosis, which may include conditions that are concerning or life threatening. Being patient-centered is critical, as the Assessment is a section into which biased judgment can often creep, manifested through specific word choices. Historically, physicians have written notes primarily intended for themselves and their colleagues only and, thus, may include diagnoses that have not been discussed with the patient face-to-face. Key components also include the clinician's summary of the plan, including diagnostic tests, therapeutic interventions, monitoring, and education. When writing notes that patients read, ideally, the plan would reflect the face-to-face discussion that occurred with the patient during the visit, and include language that conveys partnership and collaboration.

Copying and pasting the assessment and plan from hospital day after day, or one clinic visit to the next, is a common practice and can have clear benefits in time savings for the writer. However, this practice often results in an increase in overall note length, and the possibility of outdated or inaccurate information being carried forward from note to note [2], potentially leading to confusion and mistrust among

M. Isaac (✉) · S. Leyde
Division of General Internal Medicine, Department of Medicine, University of Washington, Seattle, WA, USA
e-mail: misaac@uw.edu; sleyde@uw.edu

© The Author(s), under exclusive license to Springer Nature
Switzerland AG 2023
C. J. Wong, S. L. Jackson (eds.), *The Patient-Centered Approach to Medical Note-Writing*, https://doi.org/10.1007/978-3-031-43633-8_13

patients reviewing their records. The remainder of this chapter will review the Assessment and Plan by section, exploring the challenges and opportunities in using patient-centered language throughout.

13.2 The Summary Statement

The Assessment often begins with a summary statement, especially in inpatient academic teaching settings. A summary statement is a problem representation that includes patient identifiers, key components of the subjective and objective portions of the visit record, and a likely diagnosis or syndrome. It is particularly important to consider how this statement is framed, as it may be the first line another health-care professional reads in a note, especially notes that are in APSO (Assessment, Plan, Subjective, Objective) format. Patient identifiers in one-line summary statements are further discussed in Chap. 7. There are many pitfalls that can occur if a clinician's unconscious biases are not carefully considered.

Patient identifiers should be used with caution. Labels used to describe patients can do more harm than good—though using them is customary, often they are not clinically useful. These terms include age descriptors rather than a patient's actual age (e.g., *elderly*, *middle-aged*), race, ethnicity, and language proficiency/preference. Gender identity (e.g., *man*, *woman*) may be appropriate to include, but only if gender identity has been confirmed with the patient [3]. Transgender patients report being frequently misgendered when described in the medical record, even if they were referred to correctly during the clinical visit [4]. Using neutral pronouns or gender descriptions (e.g., singular *they/them* or *person* rather than *man* or *woman*) is considered a best practice [1, 5]. Race has been inconsistently included in the past, often reflecting the provider's appraisal of a patient's race rather than the patient's actual self-identity. Given that race is a social, rather than biological, construct, its inclusion in the assessment and plan typically provides little helpful diagnostic information and can be problematic when used as an imprecise proxy for implied genetic risk.

Medical conditions (e.g., diabetes, hypertension) may be included if relevant. Care should be taken not to automatically include potentially stigmatizing diagnoses (such as substance-use disorders) or label patients as their disease (e.g., calling a patient a *diabetic* instead of a person *with diabetes*; *vasculopath* rather than a person *with a history of coronary artery disease and peripheral arterial disease*). Some terms may communicate judgment inadvertently without providing useful clinical information. For example, including the adjective "obese" in describing a patient in the problem representation likely does not convey their precise risk for cardiovascular or metabolic disease, and may not even be relevant to the presenting concern. Referring to a patient's *polysubstance* use does not indicate whether a patient might be at risk for stimulant-induced cardiomyopathy, amyloid nephropathy related to black tar heroin use, cannabis hyperemesis syndrome, or alcohol withdrawal. This sort of labeling with potentially stigmatizing information, when not necessary for clinical interpretation and reasoning, is one of the ways that patients may take offense at what they read in their medical record [6]. Keeping potentially stigmatizing information in the appropriate section of the database, and including in the assessment only if relevant for clinical reasoning for the encounter is one way to minimize potential harm.

The semantic choice to name a patient based on their disease state (e.g., *CHFer*) reduces a patient to their disease and detracts from focusing on their essential value as a human being. Utilizing "person-first" language has the potential to shape the beliefs and judgments for those reading the assessment and plan and decrease stigma [7]—e.g., "person with CHF" [5]. Notably, some communities may prefer language that leads with identity first—for example, "deaf person" though these preferences remain in evolution for both communities and individuals, so decisions related to this would ideally be led by the example set by the patient themselves. One study explored variable preferences among adolescent patients for terminology related to weight [8] and found that, while some specific terms tended to be preferred and some less so across survey respondents, preferences also were not uniform and were impacted by other factors including gender and personal weight stigma. In an effort to cultivate patient-centered language, there is potential to steer toward less precise and more wordy language, neither of which is helpful nor practical in a busy clinical practice. In addition, some language intended to be inclusive can inadvertently convey a dehumanizing tone, for example, by reducing a patient to a person with specific anatomical features, or by using terms that others feel are inclusive but may not be embraced by the individual being described [9]. Thoughtful substitutions of specific words, however, can suggest a different framing of the entire clinical interaction and therapeutic relationship as a whole. See Table 13.1 for more details of suggested substitutions.

13.3 Assessment/Plan by Problem

13.3.1 Naming Problems

One of the most powerful tools that clinicians have for making sense of a morass of complex clinical information is the working problem list; this is the structure around which the assessment and plan is typically built in outpatient charting. These topics will be briefly explored here and are discussed in more detail in Chap. 8. How we name problems depends on how much information and diagnostic certainty is available, and is also predicated on our understanding of the relationships between different presenting symptoms and known diagnoses. For example, a patient who, at their first visit, has an assessment focused on *dyspnea* may, at a subsequent visit after lab work and cardiac evaluation, then have their first problem described more specifically as *heart failure with reduced ejection fraction*.

Table 13.1 Assessment and plan—examples of named problems that are potentially stigmatizing; or nonstigmatizing but potentially misunderstood by patients

Term	Notes
Terms that are potentially stigmatizing that have patient-centered alternatives	
Morbid obesity	Use *obesity, class III*; *obesity with BMI* ___; or state the BMI alone instead
	Only list in A/P if discussed in the clinical encounter
Substance abuse	Use *substance-use disorder* instead
Polysubstance abuse	Use *substance-use disorder* instead, and note the specific substances used
Noncompliance	Address issues with adherence within the context of the medical problems instead; if important enough to address as a discrete problem in the A/P, can use a more neutral term such as *barriers to care*
High-risk behaviors	*High-risk* is sometimes used in stigmatizing manner when it comes to behavior
Failure to thrive	Describe the specific problems the patient is having instead
Mongolian spot	This is an outdated and race-based term. Congenital dermal melanocytosis is a better alternative
Medical terms that are appropriate to use, but with disparate lay meanings that may require explanation (either verbally with the patient or in the patient instructions)	
Anorexia	Decreased appetite vs. anorexia nervosa
Heart Failure with reduced Ejection Fraction (HFrEF)	The term *failure* suggests an end-stage condition and not a chronic illness
End-stage liver disease	May imply a more late-stage disease to patients than an individual's clinical situation might suggest
SOB	For shortness of breath
Positive test results	A "positive" test can be serious and have negative health implications (e.g., a positive radiology result). Similarly, a negative result is often good for a patient's prognosis
*Pseudo-*_____	Some terms such as pseudo-claudication or pseudo-dementia may be neutral to providers (one condition presenting similarly to another), but to a patient the term *pseudo* may lead them to think they are being disbelieved [6]
Senile purpura	The lay term senility has negative connotations. (Note: some use the term actinic purpura.)

Issues addressed are often listed numerically or in bulleted points in the Assessment and Plan. Because of how prominently these terms are displayed, patient-centered language here is especially important. The principles are similar to those discussed in Chap. 8.

Terms for which alternate language should be used (Table 13.1): Some terms are potentially stigmatizing to patients but fortunately have readily available alternatives that still have clinical meaning. For example, substance-use disorders have several terms that tend to be stigmatizing, including *abuse* (e.g., *tobacco abuse*, *drug abuse*, *heroin abuse*), and *polysubstance* use or abuse (lumps together substances in a manner that suggests they are the same) (see also Chap. 10). For discussions of weight and body habitus, *morbid obesity* is an unnecessarily stigmatizing term, and can be replaced by Class III obesity, or simply list the patient's body mass index (BMI). As discussed in Chap. 5 and below, obesity should be in the Assessment and Plan within the context of the patient's evaluation—that is, if the encounter was to address obesity, then having it as a problem in the Assessment and Plan is concordant, but if not discussed, then a patient will often find it surprising that it was mentioned prominently in the A/P. *Nonadherence* is a label that may appear in various locations in the chart (Chaps. 3, 4 and 7), but is sometimes called out as a separate "problem" in the A/P. It is less stigmatizing to address barriers to care in the context of specific medical conditions. If discussed separately, it is more patient centered to list the A/P item as "barriers to care" or other, more neutral terms. Once labeled as *noncompliant*, patients can have a difficult time reframing themselves to providers. Other terms that are potentially more harmful than helpful include *Failure to Thrive* (list the specific problems instead) and so-called high-risk behaviors (e.g., using *high-risk sexual behaviors* as a diagnosis for providing pre-exposure prophylaxis against HIV, rather than *Contact with and (suspected) exposure to HIV* (see Chaps. 8 and 9).

Some terms are appropriate to keep but may require patient education. The fact that patients read their notes does not mean that providers need to translate professional medical notes into lay language. Notes continue to be used primarily for medical care and communication, in contrast to direct patient education (both written and verbal) that should be tailored to a patient's health literacy. While nonstigmatizing medical jargon is appropriate, there are some terms that are nevertheless commonly misunderstood by patients. For example, clinicians commonly use the term *anorexia* to describe a symptom of decreased appetite, whereas for the lay public, the term *anorexia* is typically used to describe anorexia nervosa. Using these terms in the working problem list may be necessary for clinical clarity, but might require further discussion with patients to avoid misunderstanding and erosion of trust.

13.3.2 Disease Status

After naming the problem or condition, the status of that problem is often the next line of the Assessment and Plan, particularly for chronic conditions. Language describing the status of a condition can have varying degrees of patient-centered language (Table 13.2).

The assessment also may make note of prior treatments and a patient's response to them—for example, *patient previously failed selective serotonin reuptake inhibitors (SSRIs)* in discussing prior response to treatment. This language, while used commonly in medical records to simply indicate a lack of prior clinical response, may be read as judgmental or blaming. As an alternative, a clinician could write: *SSRIs have been tried previously but were ineffective.*

Table 13.2 Disease status descriptions

Potentially harmful language	Alternative(s)	Comment
Diabetes: poorly controlled	Diabetes: not yet at goal	Shift in language aligns provider and patient around a common goal of glycemic control
	Diabetes: Goal A1c < 7, currently 9. Discussed…	
They failed antidepressants	They previously trialed SSRIs without response/ with inadequate response	While the phrasing in the first column is common medical jargon, and may be neutral to a provider, it leaves the impression that it is the patient's fault that a treatment was ineffective [2]

In addition, describing challenges and successes in managing chronic diseases can read as judgmental both toward patients and their providers. A subspecialist writing *diabetes: poorly controlled* has the potential to convey negative judgment both toward the patient struggling at home with their glycemic control and their primary care clinician working to titrate insulin regimens. Alternatively, one might write *diabetes: not yet at goal*, which subtly aligns clinicians and patients in the effort to improve their condition. Stigma itself can negatively impact chronic disease management and clinical outcomes, as has been shown with epilepsy [10, 11] and diabetes [12, 13] among other conditions.

Certain terms are appropriate to retain (e.g., *decompensated* cirrhosis) but may merit explanation to the patient as to what it means (either verbally or in the written instructions to the patient).

13.3.3 Differences of Opinion: Doubting Language

A thorough medical evaluation includes a rigorous consideration of differential diagnoses and the available data. As such, providers may doubt aspects of a patient's history such as their self-diagnoses, attributions, and/or causal associations. Providers may also question the accuracy of data cited by other providers and/or the conclusions they draw from them. In short, doubt is critically important in preventing false assumptions and ensuring accurate diagnosis.

As we discuss in Chaps. 3 and 7, doubt can be cast in written documentation throughout a patient's chart, but especially in the History of Present Illness (HPI). Doubting language typically used in the HPI can also appear in the Assessment and Plan. The use of quotations is a common way in which doubt can be cast toward a patient's identity, context, or attributions [5]. Not all quotations are harmful; rather, thoughtful consideration of the pros and cons of including a patient's attribution in quotes versus a more clinician-centered description of their symptoms should include both considerations of which framing is most clear to clinicians, and which will convey a tone of respect for the patient. In addition to quotations, words such as *claims* or *insists* can betray underlying skepticism about a patient's history or preferences. It is a better practice not to use such language in any part of the chart.

The Assessment and Plan, however, is the most appropriate section of the chart in which to discuss differences of opinion or perspective. Rather than using terms or quotations to cast doubt, it is more useful to describe the discussion openly and address any differences frankly (examples are shown in Table 13.3). Discussion of why a clinician might use different words to describe a symptom or syndrome than a patient is best done face-to-face, and may require clarification of specific medical terms with implied pathophysiology (such as angina) and a review of the clinical features the clinician has taken into account in making their assessment.

13.3.4 Decision Making

One of the main benefits patients cite in being able to read their medical notes is the feeling of being in better control of their care, and in remembering their plan of care [14]. During a brief clinic visit, there may not be adequate time to utilize teach back or other approaches to make sure patients understand the details in both the clinician's assessment and the agreed-upon plan. In fact, data suggests that teach-back is not done often [15], for a variety of reasons, including communication challenges and limited time [15, 16]. Having a chart note, which is a reliable account of an in-person conversation, can add an additional layer of understanding for patients, and has been found to be particularly useful for patients who are older, have poorer self-reported health, and have fewer years of formal education [17, 18]. Furthermore, by conveying a discussion or negotiation with respect, this documentation can further reinforce patients' trust in their care providers. Many decisions in medicine are made in the presence of marked clinical uncertainty, or may be particularly preference-sensitive, for example, discussions around screening with a high false-positive rate, or therapeutic interventions with uncertain benefit and significant potential adverse effects. True collaboration through shared decision making in these settings is imperative, and documenting these considerations and trade-offs may further add to a patient's knowledge and empowerment.

Descriptions of a therapeutic plan should also reflect the nature of the negotiation between clinician and patient. Often, the plan proposed by the clinician may not be practical or acceptable to a patient—for example, they may not want to take a daily blood pressure medication but prefer to focus on lifestyle modification instead. As Dr. Louise Aronson writes, treatment outcomes might be better if prescribers "tailor the treatment to the patient's lifestyle, not the other way round" [19]. Careful choice of words is critical to avoid any conveyance of judgment. As has been mentioned in prior chapters, avoiding words such as "refuses" is critical, and more neutral words can be used instead, such as "declines," or "prefers to avoid."

Verb choice in the plan is especially important in conveying a more egalitarian clinician-patient relationship. Certain verb choices suggest a childlike, disobedient, petulant, or passive patient, while others convey true partnership with a treating

Table 13.3 Differences of diagnostic opinion in the assessment and plan

Less patient-centered language	Alternative(s)	Comment
"Chest pain": Patient insists it is cardiac; doubt cardiac chest pain; tried to reassure	Chest pain: We discussed that although ___ is concerned that their chest pain is from their heart, I believe that it is more likely to be from reflux because …	Example in the first column includes doubting language with the word *insists* and the use of quotation marks, which suggests skepticism in this context. One alternative is to describe the patient's view—thereby acknowledging that their view has been heard—and document the discussion of the provider's reasoning for an alternate diagnosis
Iron-deficiency anemia: Patient refuses colonoscopy despite multiple discussions re: concern for occult GI bleed	Iron-deficiency anemia: with concern for occult GI bleed. [Patient's name] and I have discussed my strong recommendation for colonoscopy at several visits. He declines at this time due to a negative experience his partner had with this procedure previously—will continue to discuss	"Refuses" is a verb, which connotes judgment. In the alternative example, more neutral language is utilized, as well as a brief explanation of the patient's perspective
Diffuse myalgias: no objective evidence of active rheumatologic/inflammatory condition. Patient adamant about getting another ANA today despite multiple prior negatives	Diffuse myalgias: no physical exam or lab evidence of active rheumatologic/inflammatory condition. Patient requests ANA—discussed today that with multiple prior negative tests, repeat ANA less likely to be useful	Slight difference in phrasing suggests an active physician-patient partnership and reflects a collaborative, in-person discussion
Chronic pain, on long-term narcotics. Patient denies using other opioids despite multiple Utox results positive for fentanyl and other opioids in addition to prescribed MS Contin. Suspect opioid use disorder	Chronic pain, on long-term opioid therapy. Recent urine drug screen results have shown prescribed MS Contin as well as other opioids including fentanyl. Patient does not report any recent use of other opioids. We discussed safety concerns today given multiple substances on the urine testing	Word choice can make a difference—e.g., "opioid" as opposed to narcotic, which is an imprecise and outdated term that may have loaded meaning and judgment for patients. The word "suspect" here may also undermine the therapeutic relationship. The alternative example reflects an in-person collaborative conversation

physician [20]. In one study, verb choices that imply doubt (e.g., *claims, insists*) were more frequently observed in notes written about Black patients. This has the potential to undermine trust and magnify health inequities associated with racism [21].

The diagnostic plan outlines the next steps required to arrive at a diagnosis. This may include laboratory or radiologic testing, or a diagnostic trial of an intervention (e.g., proton pump inhibitor trial for gastroesophageal reflux disease). The diagnostic plan should accurately reflect the in-person conversation, particularly around what diagnostic tests are forthcoming, even if the rationale for each of these is not explicitly named. In the era of Open Notes, asking a patient to go to the lab "to get some blood work done" could result in surprise and fear if they later realize that some of those tests might have uncovered stigmatized conditions (e.g., urine drug screen in the setting of substance-use disorder, HIV testing for patient with symmetric polyneuropathy), or a life-threatening condition they did not realize was on the differential diagnosis (e.g., alpha-fetoprotein levels to screen for hepatocellular carcinoma).

For situations in which a diagnostic plan is modified after discussion with a patient, care must be taken to avoid conveying judgment about why a treatment plan might have been modified. Consider the difference between *patient refused the recommended workup for his acute kidney injury despite a long and involved conversation* as opposed to *after we discussed concerns about worsening kidney function and I recommended getting blood work done today, the patient preferred to wait on additional testing due to a need to pick up their grandchildren from school.* The patient is generally in the best position to understand the competing needs and challenges in their own life. Reflecting respect for the decisions patients make, while still capturing clinical thinking and concerns, is optimal.

Similarly, challenges with regular medication use must be addressed sensitively to avoid any perception of judgment. The term *adherence* suggests that the clinician knows best and anything other than what the clinician has proposed is less optimal [22]. There may be complex reasons why a patient is not taking a medication as directed—regimen complexity, cost, and/or side effects, for example. A clinician might view a patient who has not had their medications filled as someone who is not engaged in their own health—not realizing that the patient may have to make a rational choice between purchasing their medication or paying for fundamental needs such as housing or food.

Table 13.4 summarizes language recommendations for topics commonly found in the Assessment and Plan.

13.3.5 No Surprises

In the Assessment section of a note, each listed problem is followed by an assessment, which is often quite brief in outpatient documentation. For undifferentiated symptoms, this assessment often begins with an exploration of a tailored and prioritized differential diagnosis. Included within this would be common conditions, and also more concerning (and perhaps less likely) "can't miss" diagnoses. Reading these possible diagnoses may be concerning for patients who may focus unduly on the worst-case scenario. Furthermore, clinicians may have chosen not to discuss

Table 13.4 Decision-making language in the assessment and plan

Less patient-centered language	Alternative(s)	Comment
Sinusitis: the patient is adamant that they need antibiotics for this and refuses to listen	Sinusitis: The patient would like antibiotics but I discussed with them that although previously we tended to treat sinusitis with antibiotics, clinical practice has changed over the years, and because most sinusitis is viral, antibiotics do not treat viral infections. Discussed home care, and return precautions for when we would consider antibiotics	This may indeed be longer to document, but rather than using judgmental words such as *adamant* and *refuse*, it is more useful to convey the discussion, including the differences in treatment preferences
Refuses	Declines	
	Would prefer to avoid	
	Prefers to [do alternative]	
	Requests an alternative	
	We discussed…	
He insists on not taking meds	He prefers to avoid medications	
	He remains focused on lifestyle changes primarily	
We will send the patient home with a week's worth of medicine	The patient will go home today with a week's worth of medicine	To *send* someone home implies having power over their actions, when, in reality, decisions such as these are best made in partnership
I have told him to…	We discussed…	Unilateral language conveys physician authority over a patient [23]

potentially life-threatening conditions that they have considered, but deem unlikely, in the interest of not causing undue anxiety for their patients. As such, when patients read their notes, and may see a life-threatening condition listed as a possibility, they may, in fact, be "hearing" serious news for the first time while alone and logged into a computer terminal. For this reason, consistency between verbal and written communication is essential in the era of Open Notes [6].

13.3.6 Monitoring

Explicit documentation of monitoring and surveillance for chronic conditions is another important part of a patient's plan. The rationale for monitoring and surveillance may not always be clear to patients with chronic conditions, and including a brief explanation, or language to convey a sense of the routine nature of a surveillance plan may help reduce a patient's anxiety. For example, rather than writing *incidental pulmonary nodule—will need annual CT next March*, consider the following instead: *incidental pulmonary nodule—low risk per radiology, will need annual CT next March.*

13.4 Education

All clinicians are teachers. Many of our patients come to us with little knowledge about or understanding of their complex disease processes. Speaking to issues around low health literacy with tact and respect is critical, and, while avoiding all jargon in the written medical records is neither practical nor advisable, it is good practice to remember that patients may use their records as an additional source of understanding. Patients with low health literacy use digital technology at similar rates compared with patients with higher health literacy, but tend to use different resources, for example, fewer search engines, more health-related apps, and social networking sites as sources of information [24]. Thus, the medical record may rightly be seen as another potential information source to augment the resources available to patients with lower health literacy in particular.

13.5 Conclusion

The language that clinicians use in medical documentation is deeply entrenched and reflects many of the parental hierarchies that have been part of medicine throughout its history. Furthermore, stigmatizing language in both oral and written medical culture disproportionately affects patients from historically marginalized groups [25]. The Assessment and Plan is particularly important as one of the most frequently read parts of a medical note. Now, as the tides shift toward greater autonomy for patients and a desire to shed light on some of the less ideal and outdated aspects of medical culture, our language needs to be updated as well. Language both reflects and shapes attitudes toward patients as well as clinical outcomes [26]. A more thoughtful and patient-centered approach to medical documentation is a teachable set of concepts and skills [27]. We can and should do better.

References

1. Billings JA, Stoeckle J. The clinical encounter: a guide to the medical interview and case presentation, vol. 1. 2nd ed. St. Louis: Mosby; 1999.
2. Rule A, Bedrick S, Chiang MF, Hribar MR. Length and redundancy of outpatient Progress notes across a decade at an Academic Medical Center. JAMA Netw Open. 2021;4(7):e2115334. https://doi.org/10.1001/jamanetworkopen.2021.15334.

3. Kost A, Akande T, Jones R, et al. Use of patient identifiers at the University of Washington School of Medicine: building institutional consensus to reduce bias and stigma. Fam Med. 2021;53(5):366–71. https://doi.org/10.22454/FamMed.2021.251330.
4. Alpert AB, Mehringer JE, Orta SJ, et al. Experiences of transgender people reviewing their electronic health records, a qualitative study. J Gen Intern Med. 2023;38(4):970–7. https://doi.org/10.1007/s11606-022-07671-6.
5. Healy M, Richard A, Kidia K. How to reduce stigma and bias in clinical communication: a narrative review. J Gen Intern Med. 2022;37(10):2533–40. https://doi.org/10.1007/s11606-022-07609-y.
6. Fernández L, Fossa A, Dong Z, et al. Words matter: what do patients find judgmental or offensive in outpatient notes? J Gen Intern Med. 2021;36(9):2571–8. https://doi.org/10.1007/s11606-020-06432-7.
7. Robinson SM. "Alcoholic" or "person with alcohol use disorder"? Applying person-first diagnostic terminology in the clinical domain. Subst Abus. 2017;38(1):9–14. https://doi.org/10.1080/08897077.2016.1268239.
8. Puhl RM, Himmelstein MS. Adolescent preferences for weight terminology used by health care providers. Pediatr Obes. 2018;13(9):533–40. https://doi.org/10.1111/ijpo.12275.
9. Kristof N. Inclusive or alienating? The language wars go on. The New York Times. Accessed 1 Feb 2023.
10. Blixen C, Ogede D, Briggs F, et al. Correlates of stigma in people with epilepsy. J Clin Neurol. 2020;16(3):423–32. https://doi.org/10.3988/jcn.2020.16.3.423.
11. DiIorio C, Osborne Shafer P, Letz R, Henry T, Schomer DL, Yeager K. The association of stigma with self-management and perceptions of health care among adults with epilepsy. Epilepsy Behav. 2003;4(3):259–67. https://doi.org/10.1016/s1525-5050(03)00103-3.
12. Hansen UM, Olesen K, Willaing I. Diabetes stigma and its association with diabetes outcomes: a cross-sectional study of adults with type 1 diabetes. Scand J Public Health. 2020;48(8):855–61. https://doi.org/10.1177/1403494819862941.
13. Brazeau AS, Nakhla M, Wright M, et al. Stigma and its association with glycemic control and hypoglycemia in adolescents and young adults with type 1 diabetes: cross-sectional study. J Med Internet Res. 2018;20(4):e151. https://doi.org/10.2196/jmir.9432.
14. Walker J, Leveille S, Bell S, et al. OpenNotes after 7 years: patient experiences with ongoing access to their clinicians' outpatient visit notes. J Med Internet Res. 2019;21(5):e13876. https://doi.org/10.2196/13876.
15. Feinberg I, Ogrodnick MM, Hendrick RC, Bates K, Johnson K, Wang B. Perception versus reality: the use of teach back by medical residents. Health Lit Res Pract. 2019;3(2):e117–26. https://doi.org/10.3928/24748307-20190501-01.
16. Komondor K, Choudhury R. Assessing teach-back utilization in a downtown medical center. Health Lit Res Pract. 2021;5(3):e226–32. https://doi.org/10.3928/24748307-20210719-01.
17. Bell SK, Mejilla R, Anselmo M, et al. When doctors share visit notes with patients: a study of patient and doctor perceptions of documentation errors, safety opportunities and the patient-doctor relationship. BMJ Qual Saf. 2017;26(4):262–70. https://doi.org/10.1136/bmjqs-2015-004697.
18. Hägglund M, McMillan B, Whittaker R, Blease C. Patient empowerment through online access to health records. BMJ. 2022;378:e071531. https://doi.org/10.1136/bmj-2022-071531.
19. Aronson JK. Compliance, concordance, adherence. Br J Clin Pharmacol. 2007;63(4):383–4. https://doi.org/10.1111/j.1365-2125.2007.02893.x.
20. Cox C, Fritz Z. Presenting complaint: use of language that disempowers patients. BMJ. 2022;377:e066720. https://doi.org/10.1136/bmj-2021-066720.
21. Beach MC, Saha S, Park J. Testimonial injustice: linguistic bias in the medical records of black patients and women. J Gen Intern Med. 2021;36(6):1708–14. https://doi.org/10.1007/s11606-021-06682-z.
22. Chakrabarti S. What's in a name? Compliance, adherence and concordance in chronic psychiatric disorders. World J Psychiatry. 2014;4(2):30–6. https://doi.org/10.5498/wjp.v4.i2.30.

23. Park J, Saha S, Chee B, Taylor J, Beach MC. Physician use of stigmatizing language in patient medical records. JAMA Netw Open. 2021;4(7):e2117052. https://doi.org/10.1001/jamanetworkopen.2021.17052.
24. Manganello J, Gerstner G, Pergolino K, Graham Y, Falisi A, Strogatz D. The relationship of health literacy with use of digital technology for health information: implications for public health practice. J Public Health Manag Pract. 2017;23(4):380–7. https://doi.org/10.1097/phh.0000000000000366.
25. Himmelstein G, Bates D, Zhou L. Examination of stigmatizing language in the electronic health record. JAMA Netw Open. 2022;5(1):e2144967. https://doi.org/10.1001/jamanetworkopen.2021.44967.
26. Goddu AP, O'Conor KJ, Lanzkron S, et al. Do words matter? Stigmatizing language and the transmission of bias in the medical record. J Gen Intern Med. 2018;33(5):685–91. https://doi.org/10.1007/s11606-017-4289-2.
27. Collier K, Gupta A, Vinson A. Motivating change in resident language use through narrative medicine workshops. BMC Med Educ. 2022;22(1):663. https://doi.org/10.1186/s12909-022-03721-z.

Chapter 14
Difficult Encounters

Sarah Steinkruger and Jeremiah Grams

14.1 Difficult Encounters: Definition and Epidemiology

While somewhat subjective in its definition, a difficult encounter can be thought of as a clinical interaction in which a patient or provider feels negative emotions, often as a result of personal issues unknowingly brought into the visit, or miscommunication between the patient and provider [1].

Although many health-care professionals generally assume these encounters are due to patient factors (hence the more common term "difficult patients"), difficult encounters are more commonly due to a wide variety of patient, provider, and situational factors (Table 14.1) [1]. Common patient factors include complex medical problems, psychiatric illness, ill-defined diagnoses, somatic symptoms, substance-use disorders, high utilization, socioeconomic factors, medical literacy, and strong emotions or belief systems [1]. While not always acknowledged, providers also contribute to these interactions with their own fatigue, burnout, discomfort with diagnostic uncertainty, inadequate training or communication skills, personal biases and emotions, life stressors, and insecurity regarding knowledge deficits [1]. Additionally, there are often situational factors such as language barriers, multiple stakeholders, time constraints, interruptions, limited resources, cultural differences, and variation between patient and provider agendas that make encounters difficult [1].

S. Steinkruger (✉)
Division of General Internal Medicine, Department of Medicine, University of Washington, Seattle, WA, USA
e-mail: steinkru@uw.edu

J. Grams
Seattle University, Seattle, WA, USA

© The Author(s), under exclusive license to Springer Nature Switzerland AG 2023
C. J. Wong, S. L. Jackson (eds.), *The Patient-Centered Approach to Medical Note-Writing*, https://doi.org/10.1007/978-3-031-43633-8_14

Table 14.1 Factors contributing to difficult encounters

Patient factors	Provider factors	Situational factors
Complex medical conditions	Fatigue	Language barriers
Psychiatric illness	Burnout	Multiple stakeholders
Ill-defined diagnoses	Discomfort with diagnostic uncertainty	Time constraints
Somatic symptoms	Inadequate training	Interruptions
Substance-use disorders	Inadequate communication skills	Limited resources
High utilization	Personal biases and emotions	Cultural differences
Socioeconomic status	Life stressors	Discordance between patient and provider agenda
Health literacy	Insecurity regarding knowledge deficits	
Strong emotions or belief systems		

The prevalence of difficult encounters is uncertain. Most early studies attempted to quantify the percent of difficult patients (as rated by their providers) rather than difficult encounters, with estimates between 1% and 15% [2, 3] with a higher prevalence (37%) in patients who had greater health-care utilization [4]. One study did assess prevalence of difficult encounters at a walk-in clinic and found that they comprised 18% of visits [5].

Why does this matter? In addition to their high prevalence, difficult encounters often take up a disproportionate amount of providers' time, resources, and emotional energy and cause more stress, anxiety, frustration, burnout, and even dislike of patients and use of avoidance strategies [6]. They tend to reduce provider satisfaction and empathy for patients, which can compromise a provider's ability to provide quality care [6]. They also lead to action bias as providers are more likely to simply prescribe a medication, order a diagnostic test, or place a referral, regardless of whether it is warranted, because it is the path of least resistance [6]. Difficult encounters equally leave patients feeling frustrated and dissatisfied and can reduce trust in the patient-provider relationship [6]. Patients who experience difficult encounters are less likely to follow the recommendations of their providers and more likely to have poorer health outcomes [6]. As a result, patients are more likely to seek second opinions or obtain care through emergency departments, which results in increased health-care expenses [6].

14.2 Challenges in Documentation of Difficult Encounters

While there is significant literature on how to best interact with patients during difficult encounters [7, 8], there is little formal training in medical education [9, 10], and even less on how to best document such interactions, especially in the era of Open Notes [11].

Table 14.2 Challenges in documentation of difficult encounters

Time for documentation	Less real-time charting because of need for direct eye contact and engagement with the patient
	Not feeling ready to document immediately after the visit
	Delayed charting: competing demands later in the day; difficulty remembering exact details
Content of documentation	Often longer and more detailed
	Concern for how patients or other providers will interpret the note
	Medicolegal concerns
Managing personal factors	Implicit and explicit biases
	Transference
	Countertransference

Difficult encounters may be particularly arduous to document compared to other encounters (Table 14.2). Providers often appropriately engage in more direct eye contact and interaction with a patient during a difficult encounter, thus reducing real-time charting. Because these visits are often emotionally charged, providers may not feel ready to chart the experience immediately after the visit. Delayed charting, however, leads to more work later in the day when there are additional competing demands and may cause anticipatory dread at having to relive the experience in order to complete the documentation. When ultimately documenting the encounter, providers have to balance trying to remember all the details of the interaction, managing their own emotions, recognizing their own biases, transference (a patient redirecting feelings, attitudes, or expectations about another person onto the provider), and countertransference (a provider redirecting feelings, attitudes, or expectations about another person onto the patient).

Because of the nature of these interactions, documentation often must be longer, more detailed, and more nuanced, thus taking more time than the average clinic note to make sure it is accurate. It may require more effort to remain objective and conscientious of language used. Providers may worry about how patients will perceive them based on what is written in the chart. They may fear patients reading the note and sending either complaints or edits via electronic portals that the provider must address later. However, research shows this may be less of an issue than providers fear: one study found that only 10.5% of patients reported feeling judged and/or offended by something they read in their note(s) [12]. Patients who reported poor health, unemployment, or inability to work were more likely to feel judged or offended [12]. In another study from 2020 in which patients evaluated visit notes written by their clinicians, nearly all patients (96%) reported that they understood all or nearly all of the self-selected note, with few differences by clinician type or specialty [13]. Overall, 93% agreed or somewhat agreed the note accurately described the visit, and only 6% reported something important missing from the note [13]. Again, patients reporting fair or poor health were less likely to agree that the note was accurate (88.6% vs. 94.4% of those in better health) and more likely to report something important was missing (10.5% vs. 4.9% of those in better health)

[13]. The most common suggestions for improvement related to structure and content, jargon, and accuracy. Notably though, patients who reported understanding only some or very little of the note, or found inaccuracies or omissions, were less likely to recommend the clinician to family and friends [13].

Additionally, providers may worry about what colleagues or specialists may think of the encounter or their decision making when reading the note in the future. Providers may also be worried about the legal implications of such an encounter and put more effort into documentation to protect against being sued.

14.3   Consequences of Stigmatizing Language in Difficult Encounters

Stigmatizing language may have several consequences: direct harm to the patient, effect on the patient-provider relationship, and risk of biasing subsequent readers of the chart note. These potential consequences are also discussed in Chap. 3.

When patients do feel judged and/or offended by what was written in their clinic notes, their concerns typically fell into one of three thematic domains: (1) errors and surprises, (2) labeling, and/or (3) disrespect [12]. Common errors included documenting a diagnosis that was not discussed, including physical examinations or conversations the patient felt did not happen, or that information provided by the patient was unfairly represented or omitted [12]. Patients reported feeling offended when they felt they were labeled by clinicians using descriptors such as *noncompliant*, *obese/obesity*, *elderly*, *anxious*, or descriptions of their emotional demeanor such as *pleasant* [12]. Annotations about physical examinations were also cited as sources of feeling judged, particularly when related to general appearance, dermatological or gynecological concerns, or overall physical strength and ability [12]. There was concern about possible transmission of bias: several patients worried that some value-laden labels could render their concerns to be discounted by other clinicians in the future [12]. Some patients also felt labeled by the way some notes described gender, sexuality, depression, anxiety, or their use of substances [12]. Respondents reacted negatively to language used by convention by clinicians, such as *patient claims* or *patient denies*, and particularly to phrasing that appeared to distort, dismiss, or question the validity of the patient's perspective [12]. Many felt blamed for their health conditions or felt their symptoms were disbelieved, particularly when the symptom was painful [12].

It is well known that clinician bias contributes to health-care disparities and there is now similar evidence that the language used to describe patients in electronic health records (EHRs) may reflect and perpetuate that bias. In a randomized study of two chart notes employing stigmatizing versus neutral language to describe the same hypothetical patient with sickle cell disease, they found that exposure to the stigmatizing language note was associated with more negative attitudes toward the patient and with less aggressive management of the patient's pain [14]. In a similar study, internal medicine residents diagnosed eight clinical vignettes that were the same except for the patient's behaviors (either difficult or neutral) [15]. After diagnosing each vignette, participants were asked to recall the patient's clinical findings and behaviors with the primary outcome being diagnostic accuracy scores and amount of clinical information recalled. Mean diagnostic accuracy scores were significantly lower and participants recalled fewer clinical findings (but more patient behaviors) from difficult compared to neutral patient vignettes [15].

Patient harm from reading their notes and potential biased care as a result of stigmatizing notes have not been well studied in the context of difficult encounters, but it is highly likely that difficult encounters are at greater risk of including these types of language problems.

14.4 Documentation of Difficult Encounters: Common Issues

The best practices discussed in the other chapters in this book apply especially to difficult encounters.

14.4.1 Labeling

Labeling can occur in nearly any part of a medical note, commonly found in the one-liner and history of present illness (Chap. 7), the physical exam (Chap. 12), and the assessment and plan (Chap. 13). Difficult encounters frequently become translated into negative labels or descriptors of the patient rather than the encounter. Descriptive adjectives such as *difficult, disruptive, aggressive, challenging*, or *noncompliant* can be formidable to escape and have downstream effects for future care, as immortalized in an episode of the television comedy Seinfeld. One of the characters is labeled as *difficult* during a medical appointment for declining to put on a paper gown for the doctor to examine a suspicious mole that was already clearly visible, then is unable to start anew with different doctors, because the chart label follows her. While humorous on television, this situation is often all too real for patients, many of whom may not have known such notes are in their medical charts prior to the Open Notes era or do not have EHR access [16].

Negative patient descriptions are not distributed uniformly in clinical notes, but rather are subject to biases, including racial bias. In a study in the United States, negative descriptors such as *challenging, combative, noncompliant, noncooperative*, and others were more common in clinic notes of patients classified as Black in the EHR compared to patients classified as White, with an adjusted odds ratio of 2.54 even after controlling for sociodemographic and health characteristics [17].

Other negative descriptors include such terms as *frequent flyer, drug-seeker*, and even *high-utilizer* [18]. Labels (both positive and negative, although there is likely more harm with negative labels) tend to be imprecise, rarely defined, and almost always unnecessary. For a difficult encounter, it is even more important to document facts, discuss the difficulty of a situation or encounter, but not assign that difficulty to the patient themselves.

Disease labels are discussed in Chap. 7. While some disease labels such as *diabetic* may be better defined compared to behavioral terms such as *uncooperative*, patients often do not wish to be labeled by their disease; seeing this practice in their chart note may further fray the patient-provider relationship especially after a difficult interaction.

The use of stigmatizing language can be especially impactful for patients with chronic illnesses, rare diseases, mental health disorders, or substance-use disorders. The high frequency of visits, unusual symptoms, and "complaints" of chronic pain are all often mislabeled as drug-seeking behavior or malingering, and this label can especially be perpetuated if the patient remains undiagnosed, or if the patient sees multiple specialists while searching for a diagnosis. Not only is mental health still a stigmatized topic, but surveys also point to a strong correlation between having mental illnesses and being labeled a difficult patient (see Chap. 11) [19]. Patient labels are also important in terms of evoking or perpetuating stigmatizing attitudes in the context of substance use. When reading clinical notes with the phrase *substance abuser* versus *substance-use disorder*, providers are more likely to think patients labeled as substance abuser to be personally at fault for their health issues and that punitive measures should be taken or care withheld (see Chap. 10) [20]. Regardless of whether a label may be warranted or defensible, labels can seriously harm a person's access to unbiased care. It is important to recognize and remember that labels perpetuate quickly in the EHR as much of the medical chart is copied and pasted forward without revisiting its content. Table 14.3 shows common negative labels and provides examples of stigmatizing versus neutral language.

Table 14.3 Common negative labels and alternative neutral language

Negative label	Stigmatizing language	Neutral language
Difficult or challenging	___ is a difficult patient. They refuse an interpreter but do not understand what I am communicating to them	Patient's primary language is ___, and prefers not to have an interpreter, which makes me concerned about how effectively I can communicate with them
Noncompliant	___ is a noncompliant patient who won't take his BP meds and is here again with elevated blood pressures	___ did not fill their blood pressure medication as they were concerned about the side effect of leg swelling
Substance abuser or high utilization	This is an IV drug abuser and frequent flyer who presents today again for pain meds	Patient presents today to discuss low back pain. They were seen last week and 3 days ago for this issue. They have a history of substance-use disorder and diabetes

14.4.2   *Doubt and Disagreement*

Doubt is a common feature in many difficult encounters. The provider may doubt aspects of a patient's history or disagree with their illness model or treatment ideas. The patient may doubt the provider's intent, diagnoses, and treatment recommendations. Difficult encounters in which there is disagreement about the diagnosis or treatment are particularly susceptible to negative language. For example, a study from 2021 detected more markers of disbelief in the charts of Black patients compared to those of White patients [21]. Although these words may not necessarily represent individual bias on the provider's part in every instance, they can still be interpreted by other providers in a way that could stigmatize, exacerbate biases, or lead to dismissal of the patient's concerns [21]. As discussed in Chap. 7, in general a patient's history should be documented as they relate it, without inserting language such as *claims*, *insists*, or *apparently*, which can convey a sense of doubt or even worse, sarcasm, on the part of the provider (see Chap. 3) [16]. When it comes to documentation in a chart note, the issue is not that doubt should not be conveyed, as in some situations it is completely appropriate for a provider to come to a different conclusion than a patient, but rather how conveying that doubt should be accomplished. A provider's alternative conclusions are best written in the Assessment and Plan and they should be thoughtful about the language they use (see Chap. 13).

Table 14.4 illustrates language in which doubt can be expressed in the clinician's note, but still be neutral in tone. In the HPI below, rather than using quotations and

Table 14.4 Patient-centered example of documenting doubt and disagreement using neutral language

Doubting language	Neutral language
HPI·	HPI:
Patient presents for discussion of "seizures." They claim that they had "10–20 grand-mal" seizures yesterday, with their whole body apparently shaking violently. There was a witness who apparently observed this but seemingly is not available today. They insist that these are seizures despite not having lost consciousness. They are adamant that they need disability paperwork solely for these "seizures"	Patient presents for discussion of abnormal motor movements. They had 10–20 episodes yesterday in which they had whole body shaking lasting for 1–2 min at a time. They did not lose consciousness or have incontinence or develop focal limb weakness. There were no precipitating factors. They are concerned that these episodes are seizures. They have no family history of epilepsy. They are requesting disability paperwork, because they are unable to work when these episodes occur
Assessment/plan:	Assessment/plan:
Probable pseudoseizures. Patient not amenable to hearing that these were not seizures, became angry, and would not listen to my recommendations and said they'd find a "better doctor" elsewhere. Follow-up as needed	I discussed with the patient that my clinical impression was that these were more likely to be nonepileptic seizures or spells of some other etiology rather than seizures. I tried to approach this in various ways but ultimately, they did not agree with my assessment. I provided a list of recommended next steps and asked that they consider. They indicated that they would prefer to obtain an opinion elsewhere and may follow up here if they change their mind

words such as *adamant* and *apparently*, the note writer simply describes the HPI as the patient relates it. There is appropriate space in the Assessment and Plan to discuss one's synthesis of the information and clinical impressions. In this case, the difficult encounter surrounds disagreement as to the diagnosis as well as challenging the provider's expertise. Rather than writing that the patient is *not amenable* or *angry* or that they did not listen, the provider writes their clinical impression, describes the patient's alternate view, and acknowledges they did not come to a mutual agreement or understanding. In this way both parties are heard and documented, and the situation (lack of agreement) is factually stated.

Some providers may choose to avoid documenting the difficulty of the encounter altogether, perhaps to avoid stigmatizing language but lacking training in how to address it otherwise: e.g., *Probable pseudoseizures, follow-up as needed.* However, omitting a description of the difficult encounter does not accurately capture the clinic visit.

14.4.3   Being Challenged or Accused

The example discussed above in Table 14.4 is also an example of being challenged by a patient. Often patients and providers will not agree on diagnoses, work-up recommendations, or treatment plans. Sometimes patients do not feel heard or understood by their providers. In this case, the patient identified more with the diagnosis of seizures than nonepileptic seizures or spells and preferred a second opinion. They also desired to have disability paperwork completed that the provider did not believe was currently indicated. Sometimes a compromise can be reached, but not always, depending on the therapeutic level of the relationship and efficacy of communication. In the example above, however, the patient interaction progressed past disagreement. By stating that they would seek a better doctor, the patient is challenging the skill of the provider in the current encounter. When challenged in this way, providers can become defensive or angry and this may be reflected not only in their behavior, but also in their documentation of the interaction, which can subsequently hurt patient care in the long run.

Similarly, patients can express strong emotions or advocate for their needs in a way that is not as effective as they had hoped. These sentiments can manifest as direct accusations. Sometimes accusations are severe enough to lead to termination of the clinical relationships. An accusation, whether it has any truth to it or not, will need to be documented carefully. A provider has every right to defend against an untrue accusation, without necessarily being defensive in language. Rather, it is a better practice to simply state the contents of the accusation and the provider's assessment of whether the accusation is true, and to document this in the note. For example, a common situation in which this occurs is around the issue of pain management and opioid medications as described in Table 14.5. Documenting these encounters in a way that clearly communicates the provider's treatment

Table 14.5 Patient-centered example of documenting challenges or accusations using neutral language

Challenging/accusatory language	Neutral language
HPI:	HPI:
Patient presents for follow-up of their chronic pain and oxycodone refill. Despite no new injury, they continue to say their neck and back pain is getting worse and that I do not prescribe them enough oxycodone to "really treat the pain." They demand that I increase their oxycodone dose. They are able to continue to work their job in construction. Prior MRI was unremarkable except mild osteoarthritis and remote L5 herniated disc. They say that over-the-counter analgesics "are useless and don't do anything"	Patient presents for follow-up of chronic pain and medication refill. They have significant musculoskeletal pain in their neck and low back that limits their ability to perform their job in construction. They express concern that their current dose of oxycodone is not adequately treating their pain and would like to discuss increasing the dose. They have not experienced any new injuries or trauma. No new numbness, weakness, or paresthesia. MRI spine 1 year ago demonstrated mild osteoarthritis and remote L5 herniated disc. They have not experienced adequate pain relief with over-the-counter analgesics
Assessment/plan:	Assessment/plan:
Chronic pain, unchanged, no new injury or indication for additional workup. I declined to increase their oxycodone at which time patient yelled at me accusing me of "not believing the pain is real" and that "it is because you think I'm an addict." Referrals placed for physical therapy and pain clinic. Recommended neuropathic agent but patient refused. Follow-up in 3 months	I discussed with the patient that unfortunately, opioid medications are not the most effective for treatment of chronic pain and that increasing the dose is unlikely to be beneficial in the long run. I recommended retrialing physical therapy and adding a neuropathic agent for additional management, but they would prefer not to do these treatments. They expressed frustration, stating that I do not believe their pain is real and that they believe that I am not increasing their dose because I think they have an addiction. I discussed that I do believe their pain is real, but I have a different recommendation for how to treat their pain, and that my recommendation is not due to a belief that they have a substance-use disorder. I offered to refer them for a second opinion and placed a referral to the pain clinic for additional evaluation. Follow-up in 1 month to continue discussion.
	This was a difficult conversation; I hope we were able to hear one another even if not agreeing

recommendations, while respecting the patient's desires, experience, and perspective, is important to reduce future biases and improve care outcomes.

Accusations that involve legal matters should be addressed with administrative leadership in one's clinical setting. Often documentation will then occur not in a patient's chart but in a risk management capacity; legal teams may advise on what content is or is not appropriate for a patient's medical chart.

14.4.4 Inappropriate Behavior

Sometimes providers interact with patients who actively cross boundaries or behave inappropriately. Examples may include yelling, profanity, unwanted advances, and contacting providers outside of office hours or through the provider's personal phone or social media. More severe examples may include threatening language or behavior—in those cases clinical leadership should be involved, and potentially law enforcement.

In documenting these encounters the most important strategy is to remain factual without editorializing and include as much detail as possible. It is best to avoid unnecessary descriptors such as calling a patient *belligerent*—instead, describe the concerning behavior itself. For example, if the patient is physically intimidating, document what they were doing, such as moving within inches of a provider or standing over them. When documenting that a patient is yelling or screaming, it is a good habit to replay the incident in one's mind (however difficult) to make sure to distinguish it from a patient who raises their voice appropriately in order to be heard. Take note of implicit bias before describing some patients who are more likely to be designated as hostile or yelling due to stereotyping [22].

In this chapter and other parts of this book, the problematic use of quotations is discussed. When patients are quoted in such a manner as to cast doubt, or to look down on their thought content or manner of speech, it is a potentially harmful practice and should be avoided. (Quotations can however be used to enrich a patient's voice, and some providers use them broadly and effectively, as is commonly done in psychiatry and palliative care.) For patients who engage in truly inappropriate speech, it can be helpful and important to use quotations to document the inappropriate language verbatim, especially if corrective action is anticipated. As with all quotations, they should be used thoughtfully with regard to being accurate as to the totality of the encounter.

A timeline of events should be clearly documented, including contributing factors, and all people involved. Prior behavior expectations that were addressed with the patient should be documented and cited if current behavior violates these expectations. Include a clear follow-up plan and guidelines for how future providers should interact if the patient were to return for subsequent care.

Judgment is often required, as even inappropriate behavior exists along a spectrum, to distinguish patients who are having a bad day and whose inappropriate behavior is mild and respond to corrective discussion, from those who have a repeated pattern of inappropriate behavior, or even a singular behavioral event that is severe enough to warrant action.

Table 14.6 shows an example of inappropriate behavior (yelling) and neutral versus emotionally charged language.

Table 14.6 Documenting inappropriate patient behavior

Emotionally charged language	Neutral language
HPI:	HPI:
Patient was supposed to be seen for evaluation of a cough. They were 20 min late and told very reasonably by the front desk they would need to reschedule. The patient became angry and belligerent and started screaming. They demanded to see the provider stating "This is completely unfair! You don't care about me at all. I drove all the way here. I deserve to be seen by the doctor still"	Patient was scheduled to be seen today for evaluation of a cough. Due to traffic issues, the patient was 20 min late to their appointment. When informed by the front desk that unfortunately, they would need to be rescheduled, the patient became upset, raised their voice to the point of yelling, and asked to speak with the provider
Assessment/plan:	Assessment/plan:
The front desk pulled me out of another appointment to tell the patient what they had already said. I told the patient they could schedule with another provider later in the day or go to the urgent care clinic if they really needed to be seen. The patient would not listen to reason, was hostile, and stormed out. Follow-up as needed	I was alerted of the situation and came out to speak with the patient. I reiterated what the front desk stated and explained that it is clinic policy to reschedule if a patient is more than 15 min late to a visit out of respect to other patients and their appointment times. I suggested that the patient be scheduled with another provider later in the day or go to the neighboring urgent care clinic and provided them with the contact information. I discussed that they are allowed to express their frustration, but that yelling is not an appropriate way to speak in a health-care setting. The clinic manager was notified of the situation

14.5 Best Practices for Documentation of Difficult Encounters

In addition to the common situations noted above, being well versed in common positive and negative language as described by Park et al. is advisable [23]. The authors reviewed 600 encounter notes and identified themes of positive and negative language. Notably, this is one of the few studies describing language to communicate positive attitudes toward patients in the medical record; the scope of the study did not include input from patient perspectives however. This study is further reviewed in Chap. 3.

Unfortunately, there remains little evidence-based literature to guide overall best practices, and more research into patient perspectives is still needed. In addition, as noted elsewhere in this book, language is expected to evolve over time. However, given what is known we suggest the following best practice guidelines as summarized in Table 14.7.

First and foremost, it is important to write visit notes that reflect the content of the visit and record both the patient's and provider's perspectives honestly and fairly [12]. The summary of the interaction should be as factual and objective as possible and avoid excessive use of editorialized comments [24]. Avoid dismissing patients'

Table 14.7 Best practice guidelines for documenting difficult encounters

General guidelines
• Stick to the facts—avoid editorializing or extraneous commentary that is or could be interpreted as judgmental
• Fairly represent the patient's perspective as much as your own
• Ask yourself how you would feel if this was written about you or a loved one
• Avoid openly criticizing other providers involved in the patient's care
• Do not use labels regarding race, ethnicity, gender, sexuality, or appearance, as these are rarely relevant and can communicate significant bias
• Avoid labeling patients by their medical condition
Education/knowledge
• Become familiar with typical positive and negative language (see Park et al.; Chap. 3)
• Become familiar with implicit bias
• Understand the concepts of transference and countertransference
Preparation
• If possible, avoid writing when acutely affected by a difficult encounter—take brief notes and document more carefully later
• Be especially conscious of potential biases for patients with multiple chronic conditions, substance-use disorders, chronic pain, or rare/ill-defined diagnoses
HPI/patient narrative
• Do not belittle or dismiss patient concerns; include all that the patient mentioned and document the HPI from their perspective
• Consider using direct quotes if helpful, but be careful not to come across as sarcastic or demeaning
• Include context and patient reasoning when they decline interventions or could otherwise be considered "noncompliant" with treatment recommendations
Assessment and plan
• Avoid commentary that could be interpreted as judgmental
• Clearly document the risks/benefits of any treatment discussed and next steps
Documentation requests
• Be willing to consider medical record correction requests from your patient

concerns or symptoms and make sure to include reasoning and context for why a patient may be declining provider recommendations, because context is everything [25]. Make sure to document from the patient's perspective and consider using quotations but be careful that they do not come off as sarcastic or demeaning [14]. If the encounter is still triggering, take a step back to calm down before making an entry in the patient's record [24].

Avoid openly criticizing other medical providers involved in the care of a patient [24]. Be conscious of any labels or descriptors used—ask if they are really necessary for the patient's care and consider ways they could be misinterpreted or considered judgmental by the patient or other providers [12, 13, 15–17, 19–21, 23]. Be especially careful about including descriptors regarding race, gender, sexuality, or physical appearance and ask if they are necessary to include in the medical record [14–17, 21]. Be especially thoughtful about language used for patients in poor health or with substance-use disorders, chronic pain, or rare/ill-defined diagnoses [13, 19, 20]. Remember to be consistent with documentation and not to single any one patient out. Avoid too much copying and pasting as well as overuse of templating. Minimize the use of medical jargon, acronyms, and abbreviations [13]. Be conscious of biases toward the patient as well as transference and countertransference [23]. Consider "how would I feel if this were written about me or my loved ones" as this may prompt providers to choose more strength-based language that promotes mutual engagement [12]. Avoid writing anything you would not say directly to the patient and consider letting them see what you are writing during the encounter as this prompts more patient-centered language [26]. Clearly document the risks and benefits of any treatment discussed and a clear plan for follow-up [26]. If a patient reaches out regarding corrections to their chart, consider these requests. If it is a small error, ask the patient to expand upon why it bothers them. If it is necessary, use this as an opportunity to educate the patient on why providers document the way that they do. If it is a significant error that the patient caught, amend the medical record and thank the patient for catching it.

Finally, although it is natural to want to avoid some challenging conversations, patients may benefit from direct dialogue [25]. For example, when a clinician notices signs of memory loss, the chances are high that the patient and/or family members are already worrying about these issues as well. It is appropriate to document concerns such as this in the clinical note, but best if discussed with the patient and/or family first [25].

14.5.1   SOOOAAP

One particularly useful approach to documenting difficult encounters is an adaptation of the traditional SOAP (Subjective, Objective, Assessment, Plan) note [26]. Instead of the traditional Subjective, Objective, Assessment, and Plan format, a useful tool is an expanded note using SOOOAAP or Subjective, Objective, Opinion, Options, Advice, and Agreed Plan (see Table 14.8) [26]. This format can be applied to nearly all types of medical visits and is typically more patient-centered with clearer documentation of provider thought process and a patient's informed consent.

In documenting an SOOOAAP note, the Subjective section remains essentially unchanged—it contains the patient's primary concern(s) and review of systems and often utilizes patient quotes in a positive manner to keep the focus on patient perspective and experience [26].

The Objective Section as before provides a list of measurable data, including vitals, physical exam findings, laboratory results, and imaging results [26]. It is important here to avoid judgmental, socioeconomic, or racial descriptors and to stick to objective facts [26].

The Opinion Section replaces the traditional Assessment Section of the note [26]. This is where the provider communicates what they think is most likely going on based on the data while leaving room for alternative diagnoses [26]. For example,

Table 14.8 SOOOAAP patient-centered documentation [26]

Section	Description	Example
Subjective	All of patient's concerns in their words	35-year-old patient presents with sinus congestion for the past 3 days. Has been feeling crummy and run down. This is associated with fatigue, frontal headache, sore throat, and dry cough. No fevers, chills, night sweats, ear pain, purulent nasal discharge, chest pain, or shortness of breath. No recent travel. Son was recently diagnosed with a viral upper respiratory infection. Patient does not smoke tobacco or marijuana
	Pertinent review of systems, consider using quotes if they would enhance the patient's voice	
Objective	Physical exam, labs, imaging results	BP 115/72, HR 66, RR 14, T 99.2, SpO$_2$ 98%. General: Patient is in no acute distress. HEENT: Erythematous nasal mucosa and posterior oropharynx without exudate. Normal tympanic membranes. No cervical adenopathy. Lungs clear to auscultation. Regular heart rate and rhythm
	Avoid judgmental language or descriptors	
	Only factual statements	
Opinion	The original assessment section	Most likely a viral upper respiratory infection. Differential includes bacterial sinusitis, group A streptococcus, otitis media, mononucleosis, influenza, or covid but less likely given exposures, duration of symptoms, and physical exam findings
	What the provider thinks is most likely diagnosis, but includes alternatives	
	Acknowledge diagnoses are a work in process and that testing has limitations in terms of ruling in or ruling out diagnoses	
Options	The original plan section	Diagnostics: Reviewed testing for covid as it would have implications for isolation even though he is not in a high-risk treatment group. Can do influenza testing at the same time. Could test for mono, but this would be a blood draw and currently, there are no specific treatments even if positive
	Potential treatment options and alternatives	Treatment: Reviewed conservative therapies including rest, hydration, over-the-counter cold medications, tea with honey/lemon, and throat lozenges. Okay to take supplements such as zinc, vitamin C, elderberry, or echinacea if preferred, but mixed evidence. Discussed with patient why antibiotics are not indicated for viral infection, but to monitor for worsening symptoms as some viral infections can transition into bacterial sinusitis
	Risks and benefits	
	Expected outcomes including treatments withheld or refused	
	Consider writing/dictating in front of patient	
Advice	Recommended treatment option for each concern with supportive reasoning	Diagnostics: Recommended covid and influenza testing
	Patient understanding and reasoning for declining treatment	Treatment: If covid and influenza tests are negative, recommended supportive over-the-counter therapies as above. Antibiotics not indicated at this time. If no improvement, would consider additional evaluation
	Respect informed consent	
	Consider writing/dictating in front of patient	

Table 14.8 (continued)

Section	Description	Example
Agreed plan	Summation of physician guidance and patient choice in clear statement	Diagnostics: Patient would like a covid and influenza test. Prefers not to do a monospot as it requires a blood draw
	Next steps	Treatment: Patient would like to take guaifenesin every 6 h with supplemental zinc and vitamin C. If symptoms do not improve in the next week, asked patient to come back in for recheck. If unable to get an appointment, patient counseled to send an electronic message or call the clinic. For urgent symptoms such as severe shortness of breath or fever >104, recommend going to the emergency department
	Recheck timeframe	
	How to contact regarding adverse outcomes?	
	Expected common or severe medication or other therapy side effects	

"highest suspicion for viral upper respiratory infection, possible bacterial sinusitis but less likely." This preserves an open-minded approach (especially if the clinical course changes later) and acknowledges other potential patient concerns. Remember physical examinations, laboratory results, and imaging studies are often better for ruling out diagnoses than ruling them in and diagnoses are always a work in progress. Reflecting this in documentation helps patients better understand this principle.

The Options section replaces the traditional Plan Section of the note [26]. This section includes discussing treatment options and alternatives as well as the risks and benefits of each including a review of expected outcomes if a treatment is withheld or declined [26]. It is recommended that this section be written or dictated in front of the patient, so it is more collaborative and mutually agreed upon [26]. This also offers an opportunity to identify and correct any patient misunderstandings. For example, one could document "discussed why antibiotics are not effective for treatment of viral infections" in a case in which a patient wanted a prescription that the provider did not feel was indicated.

The Advice Section, which distills the options into the recommended plan for each health concern with supportive reasoning [26]. In cases where a patient declines a treatment option, it is important to document the patient's reasoning and understanding of the repercussions of the refusal (e.g., "consistent with the patient's informed choice") [26]. Remember that even though a provider may sometimes disagree with the informed choices of competent adults, these choices must be respected.

The final section Agreed Plan synthesizes the physician guidance and the patient's choice into a clear statement the patient understands and what the next steps will be [26]. It should document interval instructions in case of changes to the patient condition (e.g., "recheck in one week if not better"), means for the patient to contact the provider in case of adverse outcomes, and documentation of any common or severe medication side effects when prescribed [26].

The elements of SOOOAAP can be adapted for a given clinical situation (in the example above, some of the negotiated options include not only treatment but also diagnostic testing). This approach helps make documentation more collaborative and more clearly separates out the reasoning of both the provider and the patient so that future readers are better informed on what happened during the interaction with less risk of communicating bias that can impact future care.

14.6   Summary

Difficult encounters are a common aspect of medicine due to a variety of factors and take up a disproportionate amount of providers' time, resources, and emotional energy while compromising providers' ability to deliver quality care by promoting action bias, damaging care relationships and seeding distrust. Improper documentation of such interactions can have significant long-term effects for patients when biased or stigmatizing language is used, whether intentional or not. Stigmatizing documentation can impact diagnostic reasoning, treatment decisions, or perpetuate racial, socioeconomic, mental health, and chronic illness biases and stereotypes. It can impact the perspectives of future providers and the quality of care that patients receive. Adopting the principles of patient-centered language may be initially challenging but is likely less challenging than the difficult encounter itself. While it may seem arduous to document difficult encounters, this chapter demonstrates that through purposeful thought and concrete approaches to writing, documenting difficult encounters does not have to be a burdensome activity. A guiding principle is to document factually and discuss the difficulty of an encounter, but not transfer blame of that difficult situation to the patient themselves. The SOOOAAP format is a useful framework to consider in order to make documenting difficult encounters more patient-centered. Remember the primary goal of documenting difficult encounters is to concisely and accurately reflect the provider's view of medical facts and diagnostic/treatment plan to future providers to promote quality care for the patient without losing the narrative of the patient and their experience [27].

References

1. Cannarella Lorenzetti R, Jacques CH, Donovan C, Cottrell S, Buck J. Managing difficult encounters: understanding physician, patient, and situational factors. Am Fam Physician. 2013;87(6):419–25.
2. Mathers N, Jones N, Hannay D. Heartsink patients: a study of their general practitioners. Br J Gen Pract. 1995;45(395):293–6.
3. Hahn SR, Kroenke K, Spitzer RL, Brody D, Williams JB, Linzer M, de Gruy FV 3rd. The difficult patient: prevalence, psychopathology, and functional impairment. J Gen Intern Med. 1996;11(1):1–8. Erratum in: J Gen Intern Med 1996;11(3):191. https://doi.org/10.1007/BF02603477.
4. Lin EH, Katon W, Von Korff M, Bush T, Lipscomb P, Russo J, Wagner E. Frustrating patients: physician and patient perspectives among distressed high users of medical services. J Gen Intern Med. 1991;6(3):241–6. https://doi.org/10.1007/BF02598969.
5. Hinchey SA, Jackson JL. A cohort study assessing difficult patient encounters in a walk-in primary care clinic, predictors and outcomes. J Gen Intern Med. 2011;26(6):588–94. https://doi.org/10.1007/s11606-010-1620-6.
6. Davies M. Managing challenging interactions with patients. BMJ. 2013;347:f4673. https://doi.org/10.1136/bmj.f4673.
7. Dudzinski DM, Timberlake D. Difficult patient encounters. Ethics in medicine. University of Washington Medicine Department of Bioethics and Humanities. 2014. https://depts.washington.edu/bhdept/ethics-medicine/bioethics-topics/detail/60. Accessed 31 Jan 2023.

8. Teo AR, Du YB, Escobar JI. How can we better manage difficult patient encounters? J Fam Pract. 2013;62(8):414–21.

9. Pluhar E, Power S, Freizinger M, Altman W. Medical education: guidelines for effective teaching of managing challenging patient encounters. Med Sci Educ. 2019;29(3):855–61. https://doi.org/10.1007/s40670-019-00729-x.

10. Steinkruger S, Grams J, Berger G. Skills for managing difficult encounters in primary care. Med Educ. 2020;54(11):1066–7. https://doi.org/10.1111/medu.14307.

11. OpenNotes—patient and clinicians on the same page. https://www.opennotes.org. Accessed 31 Jan 2023.

12. Fernandez L, Fossa A, Dong Z, Delbanco T, Elmore J, Fitzgerald P, Harcourt K, Perez J, Walker J, DesRoches C. Words matter: what do patients find judgmental or offensive in outpatient notes? J Gen Intern Med. 2021;36(9):2571–8.

13. Leveille SG, Fitzgerald P, Harcourt K, Dong Z, Bell S, O'Neill S, DesRoches C, Fernandez L, Jackson SL, Klein JW, Stametz R, Delbanco T, Walker J. Patients evaluate visit notes written by their clinicians: a mixed methods investigation. J Gen Intern Med. 2020;35(12):3510–6.

14. Goddu AP, O'Conor KJ, Lanzkron S, Saheed MO, Saha S, Peek ME, Haywood C Jr, Beach MC. Do words matter? Stigmatizing language and the transmission of bias in the medical record. J Gen Intern Med. 2018;33:685–91.

15. Mamede S, Van Gog T, Schuit SC, Van den Berge K, Van Daele PL, Bueving H, Van der Zee T, Van den Broek WW, Van Saase JL, Schmidt HG. Why patients' disruptive behaviours impair diagnostic reasoning: a randomised experiment. BMJ Qual Saf. 2017;26(1):13–8.

16. Martinez A. The harms of being labeled a 'difficult' patient. Rare Advocacy Movement. 24 May 2022. https://www.rareadvocacymovement.com/post/the-harms-of-being-labeled-a-difficult-patient. Accessed 31 Jan 2023.

17. Sun M, Oliwa T, Peek ME, Tung EL. Negative patient descriptors: documenting racial bias in the electronic health record. Health Aff. 2022;41(2):203–11.

18. Cayton H. The alienating language of health care. J R Soc Med. 2006;99(1):484.

19. Koekkoek B, van Meijel B, Hutschemaekers G. "Difficult patients" in mental health care: a review. Psychiatr Serv. 2006;57(6):795–802.

20. Kelly JF, Westerhoff CM. Does it matter how we refer to individuals with substance-related conditions? A randomized study of two commonly used terms. Int J Drug Policy. 2010;21(3):202–7.

21. Beach MC, Saha S, Park J, Taylor J, Drew P, Plank E, Cooper LA, Chee B. Testimonial injustice: linquistic bias in the medical records of black patients and women. J Gen Intern Med. 2021;36(6):1708–14.

22. Motro D, Evans JB, Ellis APJ, Benson L III. The "angry black woman" stereotype at work. Harvard Business Review. 2022. https://hbr.org/2022/01/the-angry-black-woman-stereotype-at-work. Accessed 7 May 2023.

23. Park J, Saha S, Chee B, Taylor J, Beach MC. Physician use of stigmatizing language in patient medical records. JAMA Netw Open. 2021;4(7):e2117052.

24. Davis KG, Hurd CL, Kaderka KE, Killewich LA, Monaghan O, Torrie SC, Voss-Monaghan J. Challenging patient encounters (for medical students). 2014. https://www.texmed.org/WorkArea/DownloadAsset.aspx?id=32034&usg=AOvVaw03D26-QrdK4N4-X0W8VN95. Accessed 31 Jan 2023.

25. Miralles P, DesRoches C, Brown M. Sharing clinical notes with patients a new era of transparency in medicine. 2021. https://edhub.ama-assn.org/steps-forward/module/2781026. Accessed 31 Jan 2023.

26. Teichman P. Documentation tips for reducing malpractice risk. Fam Pract Manag. 2000;7(3):29–33.

27. Kuhn T, Basch P, Barr M, Yackel T. Clinical documentation in the 21st century: executive summary of a policy position paper from the American College of Physicians. Ann Intern Med. 2015;162(4):301–3.

Part III
Other Note Types and Presentations

Chapter 15
Tests and Studies

Jessica Bender and Sara L. Jackson

15.1   Introduction

Patients' ability to view test and study results on electronic patient portals is evolving. Under the 21st Century Cures Act, immediate release of nearly all results is now required [1]. This includes autorelease of sensitive test results such as pathology, human immunodeficiency virus (HIV) and other sexually transmitted infection testing, and imaging studies, with few exceptions. As a result, patients may see their test results before the provider who ordered the test. In this chapter, we will review potential pitfalls to avoid and best practices for communicating test results via the electronic portal with patients. Best practices include discussing the test and communication plan with the patient at the time of ordering, documenting the interpretation of the results and next steps to the patient using patient-centered language, and adopting strategies for special cases such as unexpected results, sensitive results, and incidental findings.

J. Bender (✉) · S. L. Jackson
Division of General Internal Medicine, Department of Medicine, University of Washington, Seattle, WA, USA
e-mail: jessi730@uw.edu; sljack@uw.edu

© The Author(s), under exclusive license to Springer Nature Switzerland AG 2023
C. J. Wong, S. L. Jackson (eds.), *The Patient-Centered Approach to Medical Note-Writing*, https://doi.org/10.1007/978-3-031-43633-8_15

15.2   Patient Experiences Viewing Test Results

15.2.1   Positive Experiences

Patients note a long list of benefits from viewing test results on patient portals. These benefits include quick access to results, feeling more empowered, the ability to make changes in health behaviors related to results, and access to provider interpretation in an electronic message attached to the results. Many patients report access to test results is important to them and can help facilitate communication with their provider [2, 3].

In a study of COVID-19 test result receipt via a patient portal, patients expressed relief (whether the result was positive or negative), and they used the information to take action, be it informing others who may have been exposed, changing work plans, or enacting quarantine plans. Patients who tested positive still found the experience useful and empowering. Limitations of this single-center study included that this was not a diverse patient population (99% had English spoken at home) [4].

15.2.2   Negative Experiences

Patients may experience negative emotions related to reviewing abnormal test results via patient portals. Health-care providers have expressed concern about release of test results on patient portals; including CT and MRI results, pathology and radiology results, and hemoglobin A1c and cervical cancer screening results, to name a few [2, 3, 5]. Some of these concerns have been borne out in patient experience: stress, anxiety, confusion, lack of understanding of test results, lack of understanding of next steps, and increased calls, messages, and visits to develop a plan [3, 6]. In one study, 55.8% of patients with an abnormal result had a negative reaction such as feeling scared, anxious, concerned, or frustrated. Of note, 21.2% of those with a normal result also had a negative reaction; for instance, not understanding if a positive antibody result (indicating immunity) was good [6]. However, another study showed no difference in anxiety levels between patients receiving results electronically versus via other methods (such as phone call or letter), although those who received results electronically were more likely to report confusion about results [7].

For patients with lower health literacy and/or numeracy, there are additional challenges relaying and explaining results. In a study of patients' ability to interpret abnormal hemoglobin A1c results, only 38% of participants with lower numeracy and health literacy were able to determine if the result was abnormal, compared to 77% of participants with higher numeracy and health literacy [8]. If one goal of open results is for patients to be able to verify that their tests are normal or abnormal, we are not achieving this for many of our patients, and this may contribute to ongoing health disparities.

15.3 Best Practices

15.3.1 Educate About the Test and Develop a Communication Plan Beforehand

There are several ways to mitigate potential negative experiences for patients when they view test results on patient portals. The first is to make a plan about result communication at the time of ordering the test. What is the test? Why is it being ordered? How might the results affect the patient's care plan? When are results expected? How does the patient prefer to receive information about the results?

Patients are more likely to be able to interpret test results and experience fewer negative emotions if they have a full understanding of what the test is, why it was ordered, and when to expect the results [9].

Best practice habits to consider include

- **Have a conversation beforehand**. Patients who had a conversation about what to expect from test results had more positive emotions (relief, appreciation, calm) when reviewing their results. These patients also expressed less confusion about their test results and were less likely to send messages, call their doctor, or schedule extra visits [9].
- **Make a plan about how to communicate test results** at the time of ordering, acknowledging that results will be autoreleased on the patient portal. It may be helpful to estimate when results may return, especially for anticipated sensitive results such as pathology reports.
- **Consider scheduling time to discuss the result**. Many patients indicate they would rather learn about abnormal sensitive results (such as imaging studies and pathology results) from their healthcare providers instead of from an electronic portal. If this is the case, scheduling a phone call or visit to coincide with the anticipated result release will decrease patient anxiety about when they will receive the provider's interpretation and plan.

15.3.2 Address the Patient Correctly

When using an electronic patient portal, it is important to have the initial greeting to the patient written correctly. If using an automated template, it is most neutral to write *Dear [First Name] [Last Name]:* in order to not make assumptions about title (Mr./Mrs./Ms., etc.). In some electronic health records, the patient's pronouns and preferred name are recorded, but if the provider does not know the patient well (e.g., as in coverage or urgent care situations), then it is better to err on the side of not assuming the EHR data are correct [10]. See Chap. 17 for general tips on e-communication.

15.3.3 Provide Test Result Interpretation

Many of the negative experiences patient report around viewing their test results are related to a lack of interpretation. Some patient portals display results to patients in the same format as displayed to ordering providers. This may include tabular formats with long lists of tests and abbreviations, lengthy pathology reports, and medical jargon that is challenging to understand. Other patient portals have adopted more user-friendly displays that include arrows, colors, or changes in font to indicate abnormal versus normal results (Table 15.1).

Yet even in the case where electronic portals include helpful flags, patients benefit from receiving an interpretation of the results from their health-care provider [3]. This should place the result in the context of the patient's specific situation, indication for testing, and comorbidities. Table 15.2 demonstrates key elements of provider interpretations to highlight how provider context can improve patient understanding of results. The reference interval, in particular, can be problematic, as results can appear "normal" but not be healthy for a patient, or may appear to be "abnormal" but not have any health consequence for the patient (see Chap. 5 for further discussion of the concept of normality is medicine). Similarly, explanatory texts such as breast density information in mammography reports, which are intended to be helpful, can increase anxiety and warrant care team/provider explanation for some patients. Common words that patients may interpret differently than what the provider intended include *progressing*—for example, *your tumor is progressing* (patients may not recognize *progressing* as bad news); *positive*—for example, *positive antibodies* could be good to show immunity, as noted above, or *positive* findings could indicate a serious condition; and *negative*—for example, patients more frequently understood the meaning of *Your blood tests showed me that you do not have an infection in your blood* compared to *Your blood culture was negative* [11, 12].

Test interpretations should be succinct. If you find your interpretation is more than a few sentences, this should be an indication that the patient may require a phone call or visit for additional discussion.

15.3.4 Recommend Next Steps

Providing an interpretation of results is often not sufficient; providers should also communicate their recommendations for next steps [6]. Should the patient return for an office visit in 1 week, or can they return as previously planned in 3 months? Do they need medication adjustments, additional testing, or specialty referral? Are there new return precautions to review? Providers' understanding of an individual patient's anxiety level, health literacy, and capacity to handle online information will determine if the results are given in an online results note, a phone call, or an in-person visit.

Table 15.1 Elements of test results in patient portal

Test result element in patient portal	Examples	Potential benefit for patient	Potential pitfall
Actual numeric/text result	Hemoglobin A1c: 6.4%	Access to exact result	No indication that result is abnormal or normal (or at goal / not at goal)
Reference interval (a.k.a. reference range)	Hemoglobin A1c 6.4% (4.0–5.6%)	Easier to determine if their result falls within the reference range	Results outside the reference range may be interpreted as dangerous even when clinically not significant (e.g., a mild elevation in blood urea nitrogen with a normal creatinine)
			Results within the reference range may be interpreted as healthy when they are not (e.g., a PSA of 1 in a patient treated for prostate cancer whose level should be undetectable)
			Reference ranges may be inappropriate for an individual patient (e.g., hormone reference range in a patient receiving gender affirming care; racialized eGFR; patients with diabetes who have an individualized A1c goal)
Flag to indicate outside reference range	↑↓ Bolded text Different colors for normal versus abnormal	Visual cue can increase odds patients identify the test as abnormal	Does not provide context for how abnormal result is (e.g., HbA1c of 6.6% vs. 11.4%)
Trend	[↗] Other graphic trends of results	Visual cue can increase odds patients understand the test is abnormal and how it is changing over time	Does not provide context regarding how result should be changing (e.g., stably low hematocrit despite iron supplementation would be concerning)
Text interpretation	*A1c levels of 5.7–6.4% are in the prediabetes range. A1c of 6.5% or higher is in the diabetes range*	Can help patient link test result with disease process	Lengthy and confusing medical jargon may result in patient believing they have a diagnosis they do not (e.g., interpreting result as diabetes instead of prediabetes)

15.3.5 Potentially Serious or Sensitive Test Results

Potentially abnormal and sensitive results require additional care and planning. Patients often have negative experiences around the receipt of abnormal or particularly sensitive test results. Many patients express a preference to delay the release of sensitive results or to receive these results via phone or office visit [13]. As much as

Table 15.2 Helpful provider interpretation of results

Scenario	Provider interpretation[a]	Helpful elements
Worsening chronic condition	*Your hemoglobin A1c (diabetes blood test) has increased to 11%, which means your sugars have been a lot higher lately*	• Acknowledges actual test result
Hemoglobin A1c has increased from 8% to 11%		• Avoids medical jargon
		• Provides meaning of test
		• Provides context specific to the patient
Minimally abnormal result	*Your metabolic panel shows normal kidney function and potassium, which are the tests we monitor while you take lisinopril. This is good news. Some of the other tests show up as slightly outside the "normal" range but are not concerning*	• Provides meaning of test results.
A basic metabolic panel is ordered for a patient with hypertension who takes lisinopril. It is all normal besides chloride of 95 mEq/L (normal range 96–106 meq/L), which shows up as red in the patient portal		• Reminds about reason for ordering the tests
		• Assigns positive/negative label ("good news")
		• Acknowledges results that may be labeled as abnormal but are not clinically significant
Complex abnormal result	*Your bone density scan shows osteopenia, which means your bones are weaker than average, but you don't have osteoporosis (even thinner bones at higher risk for breaking) at this point*	• Provides meaning of test results
A DEXA scan is ordered for osteoporosis screening in a 65-year-old woman. The actual results are lengthy and include a T score of −1.4		• Provides definitions for medical jargon
		• Focuses on key element of results as opposed to explaining entire lengthy report

[a]These examples show only the provider interpretations; in many cases the recommended next steps should also be included (see Table 15.3)

we can attempt to plan how to communicate these results, there will be situations in which patients see results for the first time via the patient portal, sometimes before their provider has even viewed the results (Table 15.4). Many electronic health records include a notation as to whether or not a patient has viewed the result already. In the case that a patient has already viewed a sensitive abnormal test result already, it is advisable for the provider or member of the care team to reach out to the patient quickly to further discuss via phone or an expedited appointment. For clinics that frequently order potentially sensitive tests, it can be helpful to develop a system to identify and respond to abnormal results in a timely manner. For example, oncology clinics may have a dedicated nurse or other team member who reviews pathology and imaging reports daily and then confers with the provider about quickly communicating results to the patient.

Table 15.3 Helpful provider recommendations for next steps

Scenario	Provider recommendations	Helpful elements
Worsening chronic condition	*Please call the office at [###-###-####] to schedule a visit in the next 2 weeks so that we can discuss medications and treatment options. Please call right away if you become very thirsty, need to urinate more often, or feel confused*	• Provides explicit follow-up instructions with timeframe
Hemoglobin A1c has increased from 8% to 11%		• Need for more urgent appointment helps communicate severity of results
		• Lists new return precautions
Minimally abnormal result	*We do not need to make any medication changes and can follow up as planned in 3 months*	• Provides reassurance that no changes are needed
A basic metabolic panel is ordered for a patient with hypertension who takes lisinopril. It is all normal besides chloride of 95 mEq/L (normal range 96–106 meq/L), which shows up as red in the patient portal		• Acknowledges previous follow-up plan, which is unchanged (and also underscores that "abnormal" results are not clinically significant in this case)
Complex abnormal result	*Let's discuss this more at your visit next month to make a plan to keep your bones healthy. In the meantime, you can visit this website [include preferred patient education website] to learn more about osteoporosis. Please let me know if you have any questions*	• Provides additional resources for patient education
A DEXA scan is ordered for osteoporosis screening in a 65-year-old woman. The actual results are lengthy and including T score of −1.4		• Invites additional questions about a new diagnosis

If a patient has not yet viewed their results on the patient portal, providers should still use caution in communicating abnormal and sensitive test results electronically. Even if a full interpretation and clear recommendations for next steps are included, patients benefit from the additional support of a phone call or appointment. This approach applies to incidental findings as well, such as incidental thyroid nodules, adrenal nodules, pulmonary nodules, or unexpectedly abnormal blood test results. See Chap. 17 for discussion on documentation of telephone calls.

15.3.6   Patient-Centered Language in Other Tests and Studies

Patients now have access to not just the summary portion of a test result, but generally the entire report. Potentially stigmatizing language may appear elsewhere. For example, a provider's note may have patient-centered language when addressing a patient's history of injection drug use, but if the radiology referral (and hence report) states *Indication: IV drug user with fever and back pain, rule out epidural abscess*

Table 15.4 Examples of patients seeing potentially serious test results on the EHR portal prior to communication from their provider

Example	Potential negative effect on patient	Potential outcome
New diagnosis	• Lack of understanding of test result, does not realize this means they have diabetes	• Patient immediately sends electronic message to provider to ask for clarification
Hemoglobin A1c is 10%; it was checked on a routine screen for a patient without a prior diagnosis of diabetes	• Anxiety about new diagnosis	
Incidental finding	• Confusion about if test means they have lung cancer	• Patient researches results online and becomes concerned they have terminal lung cancer
CT abdomen to reassess a benign liver lesion shows a new lung nodule	• Anxiety about new diagnosis	
Sensitive results	• Worry about new cancer diagnosis and confusion about prognosis and treatment options	• Patient calls the clinic but as results were released on Friday evening, they do not receive a call back until Monday
Pathology report from lymph node biopsy shows likely papillary thyroid cancer		

As discussed in the text, these situations are often best handled by timely personal contact from the provider or clinic to the patient, either by phone or in an appointment

then that stigmatizing language (*IV drug user*) has found its way to the patient. In addition to better training and changing the overall culture of medicine, providers can assist with this by maintaining patient-first language at all times, including when writing the text that is included in radiology and other test referrals.

15.3.7 *Equitable Access to Electronic Test Results*

Patients with less health and computer literacy, and those who do not read English will not have ready access to electronic test results. Efforts to support patients with access via caregivers, patient navigators, and hands-on support with setting up passwords and technology may help to bridge this gap. Ultimately, health systems will need to continue mechanisms for test results that predated electronic health care, such as phone calls, letters, and scheduling visits to review results. Patient tracking and outreach processes must be in place when significant abnormal results arise but contact is challenged by lack of EHR portal access, phone, or housing. Proxy portal access for caregivers is another option for improving results receipt for patients who are not using portals, and the same principles of using patient-centered, nonstigmatizing language apply.

15.3.8   Provider Burnout

Transitioning to electronic documentation increased provider documentation burden. While these best practice recommendations are focused upon the patient experience of receiving the results, this customized electronic communication by the provider and/or care team requires time. Future efforts should improve the display of test results as they are generated in the laboratory, radiology reading room, and pathology department such that they are visually clearer and include key patient-centered definitions. Clinical context will need to be communicated by the ordering provider, but technologic assists, such as standard texts for incidental findings, common new diagnoses, common increasing trends (such as hemoglobin A1C or creatinine), could decrease this burden.

Even seasoned providers sometimes slip into medical language that is difficult for patients to understand. Developing standard texts that are designed with patients and at a designated literacy level could improve provider and patient communication compared to customized, labor-intensive result messages.

15.4   Summary

Immediate release of test results on patient portals has the potential to empower patients and allow them to have an increased understanding about their health. To achieve these goals, providers should plan and educate the patient at the time of ordering tests, provide test interpretations and recommendations for next steps. Special care should be taken when communicating abnormal or sensitive results, which often are best discussed via phone or via a visit with the patient. The goal and hope for the future is to provide timely responses to patients without increasing burnout of healthcare providers.

References

1. Office of the National Coordinator for Health Information Technology, US Department of Health and Human Services. 21st Century Cures Act: interoperability, information blocking, and the ONC Health IT Certification Program. Fed Regist. 2020;85(85):25642–961.
2. Henshaw D, Okawa G, Ching K, Garrido T, Qian H, Tsai J. Access to radiology reports via an online patient portal: experiences of referring physicians and patients. J Am Coll Radiol. 2015;12(6):582–6.e1. https://doi.org/10.1016/j.jacr.2015.01.015.
3. Pillemer F, Price RA, Paone S, Martich GD, Albert S, Haidari L, Updike G, Rudin R, Liu D, Mehrotra A. Direct release of test results to patients increases patient engagement and utilization of care. PloS One. 2016;11(6):e0154743. https://doi.org/10.1371/journal.pone.0154743.
4. Turer RW, DesRoches CM, Salmi L, Helmer T, Rosenbloom ST. Patient perceptions of receiving COVID-19 test results via an online patient portal: an open results survey. Appl Clin Inform. 2021;12(4):954–9. https://doi.org/10.1055/s-0041-1736221.

5. Winget M, Haji-Sheikhi F, Brown-Johnson C, Rosenthal EL, Sharp C, Buyyounouski MK, Asch SM. Electronic release of pathology and radiology results to patients: opinions and experiences of oncologists. J Oncol Pract. 2016;12(8):e792–9. https://doi.org/10.1200/JOP.2016.011098.
6. Giardina TD, Baldwin J, Nystrom DT, Sittig DF, Singh H. Patient perceptions of receiving test results via online portals: a mixed-methods study. J Am Med Inform Assoc. 2018;25(4):440–6. https://doi.org/10.1093/jamia/ocx140.
7. Mák G, Smith Fowler H, Leaver C, Hagens S, Zelmer J. The effects of web-based patient access to laboratory results in British Columbia: a patient survey on comprehension and anxiety. J Med Internet Res. 2015;17(8):e191. https://doi.org/10.2196/jmir.4350.
8. Zikmund-Fisher BJ, Exe NL, Witteman HO. Numeracy and literacy independently predict patients' ability to identify out-of-range test results. J Med Internet Res. 2014;16(8):e187. https://doi.org/10.2196/jmir.3241.
9. Christensen K, Sue VM. Viewing laboratory test results online: patients' actions and reactions. J Participat Med. 2013;5:e38.
10. Baldwin A, Dodge B, Schick VR, Light B, Scharrs PW, Herbenick D, Fortenberry JD. Transgender and genderqueer individuals' experiences with health care providers: what's working, what's not, and where do we go from here? J Health Care Poor Underserved. 2018;29(4):1300–18. https://doi.org/10.1353/hpu.2018.0097.
11. Chapman K, Abraham C, Jenkins V, Fallowfield L. Lay understanding of terms used in cancer consultations. Psychooncology. 2003;12(6):557–66. https://doi.org/10.1002/pon.673.
12. Gotlieb R, Praska C, Hendrickson MA, Marmet J, Charpentier V, Hause E, Allen KA, Lunos S, Pitt MB. Accuracy in patient understanding of common medical phrases. JAMA Netw Open. 2022;5(11):e2242972. https://doi.org/10.1001/jamanetworkopen.2022.42972.
13. Peltz-Rauchman C, Divine G, McLaren D, Park KU, Rubinfeld I, Schreiber M, Johnson CC, Allard D. Preference for immediate release of test results through a patient portal differs by demographics and type of results. J Patient Cent Res Rev. 2017;4:196–7.

Chapter 16
Oral Case Presentations

Kim O'Connor and Jennifer Wright

16.1 Introduction

The previous chapters in this book have addressed the best practices for writing medical notes that patients will read (also called "Open Notes"). This chapter addresses oral communication and its similarities and differences to the written medical note.

Like history documented in the medical record, the oral case presentation (OCP) is primarily a mechanism for communicating with other members of the health-care team. In the classic model of academic teaching hospitals and clinics, trainees (medical students, residents, and sometimes fellows) give oral case presentations "to" their attending physician, either at the bedside or apart from the patient. In the teaching setting, the oral case presentation serves many purposes: trainees convey important medical information, demonstrate their clinical reasoning, and discuss the management plan; it is the means to make sure the team has the same understanding of the patient's history and medical status so that they can move the treatment forward.

When presented at the bedside, the oral case presentation is analogous to patient-centered documentation in a medical note that the patient is expected to read: the medical team is presenting findings, analyses, and recommendations, and "sharing" them with the patient. Unlike a written note, however, formal oral case presentations are typically used in teaching settings, which vary in composition of teams, style of "rounding," and length and breadth of presentations. Additionally, with oral case presentations, the sharing of information occurs in real time in front of the patient,

K. O'Connor (✉) · J. Wright
Division of General Internal Medicine, Department of Medicine, University of Washington, Seattle, WA, USA
e-mail: koconnor@uw.edu; sonic@uw.edu

© The Author(s), under exclusive license to Springer Nature Switzerland AG 2023
C. J. Wong, S. L. Jackson (eds.), *The Patient-Centered Approach to Medical Note-Writing*, https://doi.org/10.1007/978-3-031-43633-8_16

Table 16.1 Comparison of written documentation shared with patients and oral case presentations

	Written documentation shared with patients	Oral case presentations conducted in the presence of the patient
Timing	Usually delayed until notes are finalized	Live, real time
Audience: patients	Patients typically have sole access to their EHR account	Those who accompany a patient (e.g., family member, caregiver) may participate with the patient's permission
	Patient may choose to share their notes with others; provider may not be aware	
Audience: care team	Initially, a provider note is shared with a single patient; later other care team members may read the note	Live, real-time care teams are often larger if in an academic teaching hospital (e.g., multiple trainees, attending physician, pharmacist, nurse, etc.)
Clinical setting	All	Usually training settings
Inpatient versus outpatient	Historically occurred more with outpatient clinic notes, now includes hospital notes such as discharge summaries	Historically more common in inpatient academic teaching hospitals, but also can occur in outpatient teaching clinics

unlike written notes, which typically have a delay from the time of care to finalized documentation. In the hospital setting, people who are not members of the care team are often present, including a patient's friends, family, or other caregivers. Outpatient teaching clinics may also use oral case presentations in the exam room, often with smaller numbers of medical personnel (e.g., one trainee and one attending physician with the patient and family members, caregivers, or friends) (Table 16.1).

When done well, bedside oral case presentations can have other advantages, including serving to confirm the providers' understanding of the patient's history, and as a communication tool with the patient regarding the assessment of their condition and management plan. A patient-centered approach to the oral case presentation recognizes the importance of choosing words wisely and can improve patient rapport. In contrast, an oral case presentation done without a patient-centered approach can propagate inaccurate assumptions, trigger implicit bias in the audience, and alienate patients and those who accompany them.

16.2 Bedside Presentations: Historical Trends and Barriers

Over the past century, the practice of bedside rounds in the hospital has decreased significantly [1]. There are many possibilities as to why this trend has occurred. There are numerous time pressures including the need to review large amounts of data on the computer, duty hour limitations for house staff in teaching settings, pressure to decrease lengths of stay, and burdensome documentation requirements. In addition, there may be concern that a bedside presentation could be confusing or uncomfortable for the patient. Providers may feel uncomfortable managing strong emotions when bedside discussions address sensitive or serious topics. Early

Table 16.2 Perceived barriers to bedside presentations[a]

Time pressures	• Concern that bedside presentations take longer
	• Increased competition for time
	– Larger amount of data in EHR
	– Increased documentation requirements
	– Volume of patients to take care of
	– Need to not exceed duty hours for trainees
Concern for patient well-being	• Patients may be confused by medical discussion
	• Strong emotions may be brought out by discussion of sensitive or serious topics
Psychological safety and the training environment	• Trainees may not feel safe making mistakes in front of the patient

[a]These barriers are perceived and vary in evidence; they may further vary by clinical setting

trainees may also be worried about making mistakes in their presentations. More recently, the COVID-19 pandemic has limited face-to-face interactions in order to reduce infection control and conserve protective equipment. Perceived barriers to bedside presentations are shown in Table 16.2.

16.3   Bedside Presentations: Potential Benefits

Medical literature has not found conclusive evidence that bedside presentations are superior to nonbedside presentations, although individuals studies suggest potential benefits. A systematic review did not find that patient satisfaction or understanding of their medical issues was different with bedside versus nonbedside presentations [2]. However, the quality of bedside presentations was not controlled for, and therefore, it is difficult to determine if the absence of benefit was attributable to the quality of the presentations or the location of the presentation. Several individual studies have identified potential benefits. Benefits may include a perception that the medical team is more compassionate when they had bedside presentations [3], and a perception that the medical team spent more time with patients when they had bedside presentations [4, 5]. In another study, patients reported a high level of satisfaction with bedside presentations and dissatisfaction with discussions held in the hallway [6].

There are many benefits of bedside oral case presentations that are difficult to measure, and a lack of strong evidence should not dissuade medical educators from encouraging teams to go to the bedside. The time spent with the patient should not be undervalued. In a study of interns on medicine ward teams in 2012, they only spent 12% of their time in direct patient care, approximately 8 min with each of their patients per day [7]. Presenting patients at the bedside would be expected to increase direct patient care time. Providers may also worry that patients may be overwhelmed by complex medical discussions, upset when sensitive topics are discussed, or harmed by hearing serious news in the presence of multiple medical team members. But these patient harms are not borne out in what limited data we have, and the value of learning and modeling how to have difficult conversations with patients is one of the benefits of this approach. Data supports that encounters are

Table 16.3 Possible benefits of bedside oral case presentations

• Equally efficient with more direct patient care time
• Patient appreciation of more time spent with their providers
• Perception that the medical team is more compassionate
• Modeling for learners on how to have challenging and empathic conversations with patients
• Opportunity for clarification and negotiation between patients and providers
• Higher level of patient satisfaction
• Increased provider satisfaction

more efficient when internists and surgeons convey empathy during office appointments, a benefit that likely translates to the inpatient setting as well [8]. Many clinicians report that bedside rounds reconnect them with the joy and satisfaction of practicing medicine and patient-centered communication increases joy in the workplace and decreases burnout [8]. Finally, there is concern that bedside rounds will be longer or less efficient than discussions away from the patient, but this too has not been found in the limited studies that have been performed. In a study conducted during the period 2008–09, overall rounding time was the same for teams doing bedside and nonbedside rounds [5].

In summary, there are several potential benefits of bedside oral case presentations (Table 16.3) and no clear harms, supporting the need for trainees and educators to learn the skills regarding how to do this in a patient-centered manner.

16.4 Setting the Stage

With the goal of patient and provider satisfaction and improved clinical outcomes, a move toward quality bedside presentations requires attention to a patient-centered approach.

Setting expectations upfront for bedside rounding is helpful. Acknowledging the potential benefits of learning from colleagues regarding clinical reasoning, physical exam skills, and communication strategies highlights the academic benefits of bedside rounding. Providing an opportunity for the medical team to identify concerns about the upcoming bedside encounter allows them to proactively decide how to address issues in the moment or agree to discuss later privately. Reminding the medical team to focus on "what is going on" with the patient medically but also "what matters most" to the patient aligns the team with patient goals.

16.4.1 Introductions

Hospitalized patients have very little power and autonomy—respecting their personal space goes a long way to developing a therapeutic relationship. The care team should knock and make sure they receive a response before entering a room. The care team member leading the presentation should make sure to check in with the patient regarding how they prefer to be addressed, including first name, last name, title, pronouns, and pronunciation. All members of the medical team should be introduced, including their roles in patient care. If the patient has visitors, ask the patient if they prefer their visitors to stay or step out briefly during patient care discussions. The names and roles of visitors who remain for the meeting should be asked. Minimizing distractions (e.g., closing the door for privacy, setting pagers, phones, or alarms to vibrate or silent) is respectful; sitting down rather than standing over a patient can appear less intimidating and more collegial.

16.4.2   Setting Team Expectations

As with agenda setting in the outpatient environment, it can be helpful to set expectations ahead of time. The medical team should have a shared understanding for the amount of time they plan to spend with the patient, including how that time is apportioned for the oral presentation, repeating parts of the physical examination, and direct discussion with the patient. For example, for a typical daily rounding on an inpatient medical ward at a teaching hospital, a team leader may set the following guideline: "Please spend about 5 minutes on the presentation, then we can spend an additional 10 minutes in discussion and answering patient questions. We will aim for about 15–20 minutes total in the patient room" [8]. The time spent and type of presentation may vary between location (e.g., emergency department, intensive care unit, general medical ward) and purpose (e.g., initial history and physical by a trainee, versus a "warm handoff" at bedside between clinicians).

16.4.3   Orienting the Patient to Oral Case Presentations

Importantly, the patient and visitors should be oriented to the anticipated time that will be spent with the medical team and the structure and purpose for the visit. We recommend structuring the visit in two parts: first, the bedside presentation aimed at medical providers, and second, the discussion with the patient using nonmedical jargon (Fig. 16.1). In this way, the oral presentation is analogous to the written note—its purpose is medical care and communication, and it is *shared* with the patient. It may therefore include medical terminology appropriate for accurate and efficient patient care. After the initial oral presentation, the discussion that is directly held with the patient should be in language commensurate to the patient's cognitive abilities and health literacy, and may involve shared decision-making.

For example, after appropriate introductions, the team member presenting the patient's case may explain the following to the patient, especially if it is the patient's first time in such a setting: "*I am going to present to the medical team about why you have been hospitalized. We may repeat some of your physical exam together to make sure we are seeing the same findings. We will then have a discussion. You may hear*

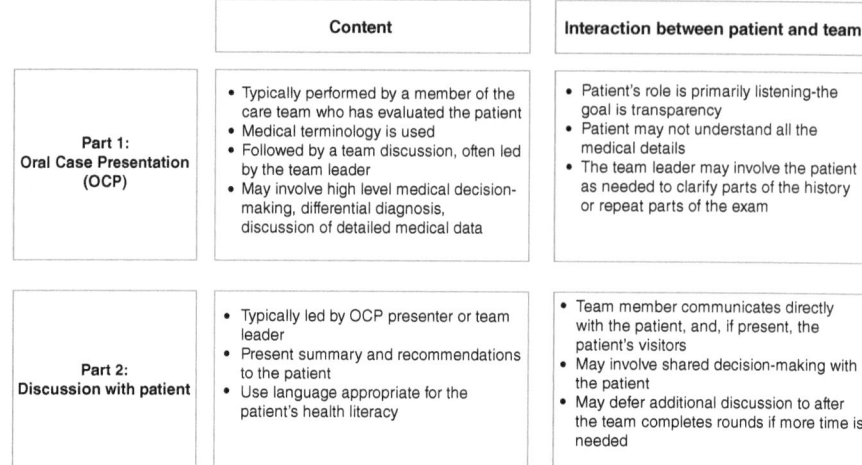

	Content	Interaction between patient and team
Part 1: Oral Case Presentation (OCP)	• Typically performed by a member of the care team who has evaluated the patient • Medical terminology is used • Followed by a team discussion, often led by the team leader • May involve high level medical decision-making, differential diagnosis, discussion of detailed medical data	• Patient's role is primarily listening-the goal is transparency • Patient may not understand all the medical details • The team leader may involve the patient as needed to clarify parts of the history or repeat parts of the exam
Part 2: Discussion with patient	• Typically led by OCP presenter or team leader • Present summary and recommendations to the patient • Use language appropriate for the patient's health literacy	• Team member communicates directly with the patient, and, if present, the patient's visitors • May involve shared decision-making with the patient • May defer additional discussion to after the team completes rounds if more time is needed

Fig. 16.1 Two-part bedside rounding

unfamiliar medical terms and that's ok—we present this way so that you can hear how we discuss your case. After that, I will summarize our recommendations for you and invite you to share clarifications or questions. We typically aim to spend ___ minutes with you, and if there's more to discuss than we can cover right now, I'll come back later to sit down with you."

The advantage of separating the "shared" part of the presentation from the directly communicated portion is that it can be challenging to continually switch back and forth during an OCP between using medical terms and nonmedical terms, or having to explain terms to the patient along the way. However, some teams engage the patient throughout the presentation; there are different styles that may work better for different care settings, team composition, and patient preferences.

Interpreted visits should be conducted similarly. In some cases, patients may not want to have the entire care team discussion interpreted but instead prefer to wait for the summary and recommendations at the end. However, it should not be assumed that they do not want to hear the case presentation and the possible back-and-forth discussion among the team.

16.5 Choosing Words Wisely: Patient-Centered Language in the Oral Case Presentation

Even though the oral case presentation is the portion of the visit that is for the medical team and may include medical jargon, there are still important reasons to uphold the principles of respectful, patient-centered language. While some medical terms are useful and respectful, other frequently used medical speech can be harmful to patients. The language we use in the electronic health record and during oral case presentations either at the bedside or privately has serious implications. Poor word choices can introduce mistrust in the physician-patient relationship and in the entire health-care system (Table 16.4).

Table 16.4 Patient-centered language in oral case presentations

	Language to avoid	Suggested language	Discussion
ID/"one-liner" (see Chap. 7)	… complaining of …	… is admitted for…	
	… with a chief complaint of …	… with concern for…	
		… to discuss…	
	___ is a [racial or ethnic identifier]	[Do not include]	Almost never relevant in the initial identification, and may bias the listener
	____ is a [language]-speaking patient here for …	[Do not include]	Language preference or proficiency may be discussed in social history; if an interpreter is used it, may be mentioned elsewhere. If an interpreter is present for the oral case presentation, they should be introduced prior to starting the meeting
	… is an elderly …	… is an 80 year old …	Age descriptors, such as young, elderly, middle-aged, are not well defined
			Use the actual age if known
	… is a diabetic…	… is a [age]-year old patient with a history of diabetes and coronary artery disease…	Avoid labeling the patient as their disease
	… is a vasculopath…		Include medical conditions deemed most relevant for the current presentation
	… is a drug user…	… with a history of substance-use disorder…	Include if relevant for the presentation; avoid label
	… is a morbidly obese patient here for …	… with a history of obesity… [include only if relevant] (See Chap. 5 for more discussion on this topic)	Outdated term
			Body habitus often is not necessary to include in the one-liner at all
	… is a 50-year-old male-to-female transgender patient here for …	[include only if relevant]	Avoid "male-to-female" or "female-to-male"; transgender status is usually not necessary in the identification statement; may be addressed later if relevant
			Encourage use of gender or sex terminology confirmed by patient

(continued)

Table 16.4 (continued)

	Language to avoid	Suggested language	Discussion
HPI (see Chap. 7)	… denies shortness of breath	… has not had shortness of breath	Could be interpreted as not believing the patient
	… claims to have not received the prescription	… did not receive the prescription	Suggests the patient could be lying
	… endorses that he has severe pain	… is in severe pain	May undervalue patient's concern
	… believes that the rash was caused by the blood pressure medication	… attributes the rash to the blood pressure medication	Suggests that patient's understanding of their condition may be incorrect
	… refused statin therapy	… declined statin therapy	Could be interpreted as implying the patient is argumentative or difficult
	… was noncompliant with a low sodium-diet	… does not follow a low-sodium diet	Implies the patient did not try to complete or agree with recommended therapy
	… describes their symptoms as, quote, the worst they've ever been	___'s symptoms are the worst they have ever had	Use of quotes, in oral presentations or written notes, could be interpreted as not believing the statement as truth
	… spiked a fever last night…	… had a fever overnight …	The term spike may sound aggressive or violent to a patient
	… no-showed to their last two appointments …	… was unable to make their last two PCP appointments because …	*No-show* implies irresponsibility; if known, can report the reason; if unknown, can state simply that they did not make the appointment rather than use the word no-show
PMH (see Chap. 8)	… end stage COPD	… stage 4 COPD with three hospitalizations this year, on continuous oxygen therapy	Implies hopelessness without clarity of condition severity
Allergies and adverse reactions to medications	… azithromycin is listed but is not a real allergy…	… had nausea and diarrhea from azithromycin…	A patient may refer to a nonallergic reaction to a medication colloquially as an allergy; if it is only acknowledged as not being *real*, then the patient's experience is not validated. Describing the reaction is more useful; can address later whether to take that reaction into account, if needed

Table 16.4 (continued)

	Language to avoid	Suggested language	Discussion
Family history	Family history is unremarkable	Family history is noncontributory	
Social history (see Chap. 9)	… is homeless…	… lives in their van or stays with a friend …	Many different terms exist for not having stable housing; if using a term, check with the patient first. Or describe living situation rather than using a label
	… is unemployed…	… previously worked in retail, currently not working …	May add details if known; avoid "unemployed" label
Health-related behaviors (see Chap. 10)	… illicit drugs: none…		Use patient-first language to describe substance-use disorders
	…history of tobacco abuse…	Smoked 1 pack per day for 10 years, quit 2 years ago	Use objective data of substances used
PE (see Chap. 12)	… disheveled …	[Leave out]	Grooming is generally unnecessary as an exam finding
	… pleasant…	[Leave out]	Descriptions about attitude, race, ethnicity are not objective exam findings
	… elderly …	[Leave out]	As with the ID, appearance of age is generally not objective
	… obese …	[Leave out]	Body mass index will be known from objective data; if specific aspects of body habitus are relevant, can report in the appropriate section of the exam
A/P	… chills overnight but didn't have a real fever …	Fever to 100F overnight did not meet our threshold to draw cultures…	Calling a lower-grade fever not *real* diminishes the patient's experience; the true meaning is that it did not meet a threshold to evaluate further
	… we can send them home if they pass a road test this morning …	… stable medically for discharge, but should be evaluated by PT to make sure they are able to go home safely…	Avoid medical slang
	… awaiting placement …	… awaiting a bed at a rehab facility …	Placement implies a lack of agency on the patient's part
	… failed first-line therapy…	… first-line therapy was not successful…	Attributes failure in treatment to the patient

ID identification, *HPI* history of present illness, *PMH* past medical history, *A/P* assessment and plan

Unlike a written note that a patient reads later, the oral case presentation has the advantage of being able to observe the reactions of a patient and their visitors in real time. The presenter and team members should pay attention to a patient's verbal and physical cues—if there appears to be a strong reaction to something said, the presenter can pause their presentation to check in with the patient: "*Let me pause a moment, [addressing the patient directly] ____, what did I miss in describing your chest pain?*"

Recognize that some medical terms or medical conditions may be misunderstood by patients or feel hurtful. If possible, consider including a brief explanation of the term to the patient early on in your presentation to decrease potential harm. For example, consider saying *hepatitis due to alcohol use* versus *alcoholic hepatitis* or *breathing problems related to your weight, which we refer to as obesity hypoventilation syndrome*, or *decreased functioning of your heart, which we call heart failure*. If you did not predict that a term would be hurtful, and you notice a reaction from the patient, this is the time to pause and explain your language. In addition, there may be terms that even after explanation, the provider realizes could still be improved. Recognizing when patients find language to be problematic and partnering with them may be a way to advocate for positive changes in language. Just as *morbid obesity* and *geriatric pregnancy* (patients over age 35) are outdated now, there may be current terms that merit reconsideration.

16.5.1   Identification and Labels: The "One-Liner"

The one-liner is critically important as the first part of the OCP that the patient hears in real time. Unlike a written note, if language is used early in the presentation that is potentially harmful to the patient, it can damage rapport for the remainder of the meeting if not recognized and addressed. With this in mind, person-first rather than identity-first language is preferred in most cases. ____ *is a patient with diabetes* suggests that the person is impacted by the illness but ____ *is a diabetic* suggests that they are no more than the disease. Labels such as *drug use*," *drug abuser*, *smoker*, *vasculopath*, and *noncompliant*" should also be avoided. In most cases, assigned sex at birth, sexual orientation or sexual practices, disability status, body size, race, ethnicity, and language proficiency do not belong in an identifying first line of a presentation with the purpose of introducing a patient. The reason for the hospitalization or visit is relevant, along with selected medical conditions. Chapter 7 discusses this topic in more detail.

Other medical slang may find its way into oral discussions that providers may know to avoid in written documentation. References to a patient's utilization such as *frequent flyer* (a patient with a history of frequent hospitalizations) and *bounce-back* (a patient readmitted within a short period of time to the same hospital team that took care of them previously) should be discouraged [9]. With speech, there is not the opportunity to edit before finalizing as there is in an EHR note; ideally eliminating the routine, habitual use of such language will make it less likely to arise during case presentations and discussions in front of patients.

16.5.2   The History of Present Illness and Review of Systems

When presenting the HPI in front of the patient, it is an opportunity to show that the patient has been heard and their story represented faithfully. The patient should feel supported and heard in the care environment, therefore descriptive language should be objective when possible. Traditional terms such as *claims* or *denies* may seem benign to providers but may cast doubt (intentionally or unintentionally) on the patient's experience. In addition, focusing on factual or objective data may help avoid bias. The HPI and ROS are discussed further in Chaps. 7 and 12.

16.5.3   Past Medical History, Social History, Family History, and Habits

Language can be particularly stigmatizing when addressing certain conditions such as substance-use disorder, chronic pain, and obesity. The use of certain terms can further perpetuate bias and imply that a patient is no more than their disease. In one RCT of over 500 mental health providers, when providers were presented with two vignettes one of which used the term *substance abuser* and the other using the term *patient with substance-use disorder*, the use of the term *substance abuser* significantly increased the provider's sense that the person deserved blame and punishment for their condition [10]. Language can implicitly blame the patient for their medical conditions rather than recognizing that social, structural, and other contributors often drive unhealthy behavior. Acknowledging these obstacles in the history rather than criticizing the patient can establish a more therapeutic relationship.

Some terms had official medical definitions but are now outdated (e.g., *morbid obesity*). Others may have current, proper medical meaning but may be alarming to patients—for example, *heart failure* may include a wide range of severity—the term may have to be explained later to the patient in the context of their own disease severity, especially for patients who have mild disease with a good prognosis.

These topics are discussed further in Chaps. 8, 9, and 10.

16.5.4   The Physical Exam

The oral presentation of the physical exam may be particularly problematic if it includes language that is unnecessarily upsetting to a patient. As discussed in Chap. 12, general descriptors often lack objectivity or clear definitions. These may include terms about age (e.g., *elderly* or *appears older than stated age*), race or ethnicity (social constructs and not objective physical findings), and body habitus (e.g., *obese* may be factually true by body mass index definitions, but as a general descriptor typically does not add value). Terms relating to demeanor, whether positive (e.g., *pleasant*) or negative (e.g., *uncooperative*) may be used in a biased fashion and often do not add to the medical evaluation. It is also important to recognize the possibility of unintentionally blaming the patient if an exam is difficult—for example, stating that jugular venous pressure was unable to be assessed due to body habitus (see Chap. 5).

16.5.5   The Assessment and Plan

If the OCP presenter summarizes the case with a one-liner, the same principles apply as with the initial one-line identification with regard to being considerate as to what details should be in that one-line identifying statement.

The oral case presentation conducted in front of a patient is not necessarily easy or intuitive—rather, it is a skill. For example, in the 2-part format, it is challenging to give a presentation in front of a patient in which the patient is not initially an active part of the discussion, but at the same time maintain a patient's agency. During the Assessment and Plan in particular, as the team discusses possibilities for differential diagnosis, testing, and treatment, language can affect how the patient is discussed. For example, saying *"I recommend an urgent endoscopy to find the source of the patient's GI bleed"* still uses some jargon (GI bleed) but is different than saying *"We need to call GI and get this patient scoped today"* (speaks about the patient undergoing an invasive procedure as if the patient is an object).

Other medical slang should be avoided. For example, if a patient's medical conditions have stabilized but the team is uncertain if they are strong enough to go home, saying *"I'd like to consult PT to see if they are strong enough to walk safely"* is preferable to saying *"We can send them home if they pass a road test this morning"* (paternalistic use of the word *send* as well as the phrase *road test* makes the patient sound like someone with no agency). Medical slang likely varies by location and can change over time—while not all medical slang is derogatory or problematic, in general, for an oral case presentation conducted in front of a patient, it is generally inappropriate and the medical team should uphold professionalism in speech.

In contrast to assigning a patient less agency than they should have, other terms in the Assessment and Plan often attribute to the patient more agency than they might actually possess. For example, saying that a patient *"failed"* treatment often has more to say about the treatment failing the patient rather than the other way around.

Potentially serious diagnoses or prognoses: One challenge unique to the bedside presentation is if a new serious diagnosis or prognosis is discussed in the oral case presentation or ensuing team discussion without the patient being able to prepare for it psychologically. If a potentially serious diagnosis is but one of a long list of potential differential diagnoses as the team is working through an unknown case, then the team may inform the patient ahead of time as follows: *"We will be discussing many possible diagnoses—they may range in how serious they are—we will let you know right away if any of the more serious ones are likely."* However, if there is a significant and highly likely or certain new serious diagnosis, that discussion is better done apart from the oral case presentation, typically in a separate meeting with the patient with a smaller number of team members. For example, if the results of a CT scan returned in the afternoon and they are highly suspicious for cancer, a member of the care team should sit down with the patient that same day, rather than presenting the findings at morning rounds for the first time.

16.6 Ending the Visit

As with any visit, ensuring patient understanding and agreement with diagnostic and treatment plans improves adherence and patient satisfaction [11]. Summary statements for the patient should be clear and concise and use nonmedical language. If necessary, clarify any medical jargon used. Small amounts of information should be shared with frequent check-ins providing the opportunity to check for patient understanding, questions, and concerns. Avoid the tendency to download large quantities of information all at once. Utilizing the "teach back" method is a proven approach to assess understanding. *"We have discussed a lot of information today. Just to make sure that I explained things clearly, can you let me know your understanding of what we discussed?"* Ending the encounter with *"What questions or concerns do you have?"* (rather than *"Do you have any questions?"*) suggests it is okay to have questions and invites patients or visitors to share their thoughts without feeling guilty, uneducated, or burdensome. Finally, provide support and acknowledgement that this is a partnership, and you look forward to continued conversations about their care.

16.7 Other Types of Oral Presentations

For the provider team, there may be occasions when conducting oral case presentations without the patient or family members present is indicated. This may be the case when complicated care discussions need to occur between multiple providers and consensus agreed upon before discussing with the patient. Patients may be altered or confused and unable to participate in a meeting with the medical team—hearing an oral case presentation if they have delirium may be further upsetting to the patient rather than valuable. When presentations occur not in front of the patient, ensure that the discussions are held in private (i.e., not in a public hallway) in order to protect patient confidentiality.

Additionally, we favor continuing to use the principles of patient-centered language *whether the patient is present or not*. Language becomes habitual, and the more often health-care professionals use patient-centered language throughout their discourse, the more likely they will use that language in front of the patient. Using more respectful language may mitigate overall bias in health-care settings and reduce some of the negative effects of the "hidden curriculum" [12].

In addition to oral case presentations, there are other times when health-care professionals present patient information to each other verbally with the patient present. For example, multidisciplinary rounds in the hospital may be led by the patient's bedside nurse (this model is often employed in intensive care unit settings) rather than a trainee, physician, or another provider. Handoffs may occur at bedside between members of the care team in the presence of the patient (e.g., a nurse at change of shift, or a direct handoff between providers for a seriously ill patient). Different members of the care team may have discussions with the patient present as well (e.g., a nurse and physician, or a physical therapist and nurse practitioner). While these other types of communication are less well studied, they would also benefit from patient-centered language.

16.8 Conclusion

The language that we use when discussing patients has evolved over time and will continue to do so. These changes have largely focused on being more patient-centered and have aimed to mitigate the bias and racism that exists in medicine. In addition to strengthening therapeutic relationships, it is hoped that these changes in language will result in similar positive changes in the culture of medicine.

References

1. Stickrath C, Noble M, Prochazka A, et al. Attending rounds in the current era: what is and is not happening. JAMA Intern Med. 2013;173(12):1084–9.
2. Gamp M, Becker C, Tondorf T, et al. Effect of bedside vs. non-bedside patient case presentation during Ward rounds: a systematic review and meta-analysis. J Gen Intern Med. 2019;34(3):447–57.
3. Ramirez J, Singh J, Williams AA. Patient satisfaction with bedside teaching rounds compared with nonbedside rounds. South Med J. 2016;109(2):112–5.
4. Lehmann LS, Brancati FL, Chen MC, Roter D, Dobs AS. The effect of bedside case presentations on patients' perceptions of their medical care. N Engl J Med. 1997;336(16):1150–5.
5. Gonzalo JD, Chuang CH, Huang G, Smith C. The return of bedside rounds: an educational intervention. J Gen Intern Med. 2010;25(8):792–8.
6. Wang-Cheng RM, Barnas GP, Sigmann P, Riendl PA, Young MJ. Bedside case presentations: why patients like them but learners don't. J Gen Intern Med. 1989;4(4):284–7.
7. Block L, Habicht R, Wu AW, et al. In the wake of the 2003 and 2011 duty hours regulations, how do internal medicine interns spend their time? J Gen Intern Med. 2013;28(8):1042–7.
8. Lichstein PR, Atkinson HH. Patient-centered bedside rounds and the clinical examination. Med Clin North Am. 2018;102(3):509–19.
9. Goldman B. Derogatory slang in the hospital setting. AMA J Ethics. 2015;17(2):167–71. https://doi.org/10.1001/virtualmentor.2015.17.2.msoc2-1502.
10. Kelly JF, Westerhoff CM. Does it matter how we refer to individuals with substance-related conditions? A randomized study of two commonly used terms. Int J Drug Policy. 2010;21(3):202–7.

11. Fortin AH 6th. Communication skills to improve patient satisfaction and quality of care. Ethn Dis. 2002;12(4):S3-58-61.
12. Lehmann LS, Sulmasy LS, Desai S, ACP Ethics, Professionalism and Human Rights Committee. Hidden curricula, ethics, and professionalism: optimizing clinical learning environments in becoming and being a physician: a position paper of the American College of Physicians. Ann Intern Med. 2018;168(7):506–8. https://doi.org/10.7326/M17-2058.

Chapter 17
Care Outside of the Clinical Encounter: Electronic Communications and Documentation of Telephone Calls

Jennifer Wright and Kim O'Connor

17.1 Introduction

High-quality, patient-centered care requires effective and timely communication between clinicians and patients. With the rapid increase in the use of electronic health records (EHRs), the modes of communication between patients and their health-care teams outside of in-person appointments have evolved.

While phone calls have long been used to communicate between patients and their health-care teams, the EHR allows for additional options for electronic communication. Furthermore, these forms of communication and documentation are now increasingly visible to the patient as they access their chart in the EHR portal. In this chapter, we address best practices in documenting these different types of communication.

In particular, the use of electronic communication (e-communication) has increased dramatically, including a 157% increase in messaging during the COVID-19 pandemic that has not diminished [1, 2]. E-communications include secure messaging (either via a telephone-based text message or a separate mobile phone application), emails (through standard email vendors), or EHR-based messaging (essentially emails via the EHR, but within the security of the EHR system). The purposes of e-communications are vast, overlap with the reason for phone calls, and often include scheduling appointments, reviewing test/study results, locating records, reviewing chart notes, requesting refills, paperwork requests, and addressing specific health questions. In this chapter, we will primarily address the patient-centered language that is saved in a patient's EHR (EHR-based messaging).

J. Wright (✉) · K. O'Connor
Division of General Internal Medicine, Department of Medicine, University of Washington, Seattle, WA, USA
e-mail: sonic@uw.edu; koconnor@uw.edu

© The Author(s), under exclusive license to Springer Nature Switzerland AG 2023
C. J. Wong, S. L. Jackson (eds.), *The Patient-Centered Approach to Medical Note-Writing*, https://doi.org/10.1007/978-3-031-43633-8_17

In some EHR systems, patient care is grouped into "encounters" such as a clinic visit, or a phone call encounter, or a hospital admission. In many cases, a single encounter may include all types of patient communications. For example, a patient may send an EHR-based message ahead of an outpatient clinic appointment, then be seen in the office visit where a provider enters a note, and then the provider may document a follow-up phone conversation about a test result later that day, all within the same EHR encounter. Knowing best practices for using patient-centered language in documentation in all these settings is an important part of being facile with increasingly complex modes of clinical care.

17.2 Electronic Communication: Patterns of Use

17.2.1 Prevalence

In a large study using data from 2019 (5438 responders) assessing American patients' use of e-communication with clinicians over the past 12 months, the overall prevalence was 60.3%, which increased from 7% in 2003 and 31.5% in 2014 (Fig. 17.1) [3].

17.2.2 Disparities

Despite the increase in overall use, 83% of this use occurred in patients younger than age 65, a proportion relatively unchanged compared to 2003. Individuals who are female, with higher education, higher income, more comorbidities, and those living in nonrural areas more often use e-communication [3]. Utilization also appears higher in academic centers, larger practices, and primary care [4]. In 2020, in a study of a diverse patient population in Nebraska, after adjustment for age, sex, education, and income, race/ethnicity was not associated with patients accessing the patient portal. However, White patients were more frequently offered access [5]. Patients with lower health literacy are also less likely to use health information technology [6].

Fig. 17.1 Increasing prevalence of e-communication between patients and clinicians in the United States. (Data from Yang et al. JMIR 2022 [3])

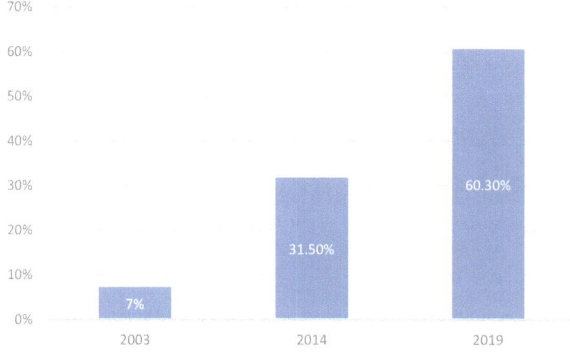

17.2.3 *Improving Equity*

Given the numerous factors contributing to the growing digital divide, there is much work to be done to make access to e-communication more equitable. One strategy that has been successful is in-person enrollment and training for patients on how to use patient portals [7]. For older patients and non-English-speaking patients, asking if they have trusted friends or family members who could be given proxy-access to their EHRs may help overcome this divide as well.

As e-communication use increases, attention should be focused on potential gaps in communication, patient safety issues, and confidentiality [4]. We must also recognize and address disparities and barriers in e-communication use by socially disadvantaged populations.

17.3 Benefits and Drawbacks of E-Communication

E-communication has both potential benefits as well as drawbacks (Table 17.1).

There is limited evidence on the impacts on patient satisfaction and health outcomes related to patient portals and e-communication, but available studies suggest that it may enhance the doctor-patient relationship, improve health status awareness, and increase adherence to therapy. Whether it improves health-care utilization and efficiency is less clear [8, 9]. There is also some evidence that e-communication use is associated with better perceived quality of care by patients [3].

Although the majority of patients appear enthusiastic about the use of this mode of communication, there are differing opinions among providers. The time spent attending to messages in the EHR has been linked to physician burnout [10]. There is further evidence that this workload is not distributed equally; for example, female providers receive more patient and staff messages than male providers, potentially contributing to higher rates of burnout in female providers [11].

In addition, as discussed above, as health systems move toward a default of e-communication, many patients will be at risk of being left behind. Assuring that phone and mail communication routes are maintained is important. Systems that

Table 17.1 Potential benefits and drawbacks of e-communication for patient care

Potential benefits	Potential drawbacks
• Improve patient awareness of their health status, medications	• Increased patient questions between clinic visits, increasing workload for providers and clinic staff
• Patients able to message providers and clinic outside of office hours	• Technology not available to all patients
• Improved efficiency of patient scheduling and refill requests	• Not accessible to non-English speakers
• Automation of lab result communication (see Chap. 15)	

safeguard that electronic messages are received and read should be strongly considered. Otherwise, when patients change their email address or lose their access to an electronic device, this communication method can break down.

17.4 Recommendations for Patient-Provider Electronic Communication

Since electronic communication is here to stay, it is important to learn approaches to this form of communication that enhances patient-provider relationships, improves clinical outcomes, and increases patient satisfaction. But these valuable goals need to be balanced to prevent provider burnout.

The majority of patients utilize patient portals; however, some providers also communicate via email, text-messaging, and messaging applications. Due to HIPAA (Health Insurance Portability and Accountability Act) compliance rules, the preferred method of communication when available is via a patient portal directly connected to the patient chart. Whenever possible, re-direct patients who reach out via email to the secure patient portal.

In general, e-communication should enhance an already established patient-provider relationship but should not replace in-person communication. Proven patient-centered communication skills such as open-ended questions, active listening, eye contact, physical exam, frequent summarization, and discussion do not translate well to e-communication encounters and are important to building therapeutic relationships. The absence of in-person contact, where providers can monitor patient understanding through verbal and nonverbal cues, may increase the risk of misunderstandings and miscommunications. A small study analyzing patient-portal messaging between patients and health-care professionals found that more than half of the replies sent by health-care professionals lacked supportive talk and partnership building [12]. Maintaining in-person relationships and the use of empathic, patient-centered e-communication techniques may help mitigate this. Best practices are shown in Table 17.2.

Table 17.2 Summary of best practices in e-communication

Before initiation of e-communication	• Establish an in-person relationship
	• Discuss risks, benefits, and expectations of appropriate use
Upon receipt of e-communication	• Acknowledge receiving the communication and the expected time for a response (consider an automated response unique to your practice environment)
When composing the response	• If it is not your patient (e.g., in cross-coverage situations), introduce yourself
	• Keep response brief and avoid jargon or medical terminology
	• Provide the patient with information on the next steps
	• Aim to keep a friendly tone

17.4.1   Setting the Stage for Success in E-Communications

In order to ensure more equal access for patients, it is a best practice to offer all patients access to the patient portal. If accepted, the next important step is to discuss expectations. Although practices will vary by institution, Table 17.3 offers some common components to consider.

Table 17.3 Issues to include in initial discussion with patients

E-communication topic	Examples (may vary by practice)
• Requests best suited to the patient portal	• Scheduling appointments
	• Routine refills of medications that are not controlled substances
	• Brief focused follow-up as negotiated during recent clinic visit
• Requests that are not best addressed in the patient portal	• Advice regarding new symptoms
	• Requests to start a new medication
	• Request for complicated testing or referrals if not already discussed
	• Request to fill out complicated paperwork
• Explanation of how messages are handled	• Hours during which messages are reviewed
	• Expected timeframe for a response
	• The team member(s) who review the messages and may respond to the patient
• Handling of test results (see Chap. 15)	• There may be a difference in timing between when results are released through the portal and if/when the ordering provider comments on those results to the patient
	• Some health systems release results online as soon as they are finalized ("autorelease")
	• If a provider comments on or takes action on results, advise the patient of the time frame in which they can expect this to occur
• Patient confidentiality	• Patients are expected to use their own chart only
	• If a patient's family members are cared for in the same health-care system, they should only send messages about the patient in the chart of that same patient (e.g., do not send a message about a spouse in one's own EHR chart; instead, the spouse should send a message in their own EHR account)
	• If others are communicating on behalf of the patient, encourage them to sign up as official proxies in the patient's EHR portal if possible, and identify themselves when writing via e-communication
• Risks of e-communication	• E-communication does not replace an in-person or telemedicine evaluation
	• E-communication is not appropriate for urgent health issues

Table 17.4 Examples of patient follow-up ideal for e-communication after a clinic appointment

Scenario	Clear patient instructions during the clinic appointment
A patient was started on a blood pressure medication and will be checking their home blood pressure readings	Please send me a message with your home blood pressure readings in 2 weeks. If they are still elevated, I will increase your medication dose.
A patient with knee pain due to osteoarthritis	We can start with diclofenac gel and physical therapy, but if your symptoms don't improve after 6 weeks of physical therapy, please let me know, and I can refer you to see an orthopedic specialist.

17.4.2   Anticipate and Prepare Patients for E-Communication Follow Up

There are some patient care issues that may be well suited to e-communication. These include planned and straightforward follow up. When concluding the visit, it is best to provide clear instructions regarding how the patient will be expected to use e-communication after an appointment (Table 17.4).

In contrast, a new health-care concern can rarely be adequately addressed in an e-communication compared to an office visit.

17.4.3   Responding to E-Communications

There are several interventions that can improve e-communication responses to the patient.

When messages are initially received, it is ideal to have an automatic response to the patient reminding them of the expected time frame for a response and what to do if they feel the issue is urgent and requires more timely attention. This should decrease possible frustration regarding the timeliness of a response.

When composing an e-communication to a patient, there are similarities and differences between direct e-communication and sharing medical notes. With medical notes, the primary purpose is to document the clinical encounter and provide care information for the next health-care professional who reads the note. Jargon may be used, and it is not expected that a patient will understand every medical detail. E-communications, however, are more similar to direct patient counseling or written patient instructions. E-communications should be written at a level the patient can understand. However, a challenge with e-communications is the one-sided nature of the communication and the potential for misinterpretation of language and tone (Table 17.5).

Table 17.5 Comparison of in-person visits, e-communications, and sharing of medical notes

Topic	In-person appointment between patient and provider	Medical note shared with the patient	E-communication (e.g., messages in the EHR between patient and provider)
Purpose	• Patient care	• Clinical documentation	• Direct communication with patient • May also serve as documentation
Patient-centered language	• Should be used	• Should be used	• Should be used
Medical Jargon	• Should be avoided, or adjusted based on the patient's health literacy	• May be used as appropriate	• Should be avoided, or adjusted based on the patient's health literacy
Interaction	• Immediate, real time	• Delayed. Unless the note is cowritten (this is rare), the note is completed after a visit and patient reads the shared note later	• May involve back-and-forth communication (replying to messages)
	• Can assess and respond to nonverbal cues and provide immediate clarification	• Typically no back-and-forth communication	• Usually not real time, but may have minimal delay to several days depending on patient and provider factors • Increased potential for miscommunication in language or tone

Some concerns may be readily addressed by e-communication, although feasibility will also depend on a provider's or staff member's time allocated to responding to messages. Anticipating the next steps may assist with reducing further e-communications from patients (Table 17.6).

In the example in Table 17.6, the patient's blood pressure medication is adjusted over an EHR message. Since this is not a new medication, and presumably the provider and patient have already reviewed potential side effects to watch for, the provider felt comfortable making this adjustment without an appointment. However, the provider also sets up the next step—recommending an appointment to follow up and includes a time frame. For the patient with respiratory symptoms, the provider provides recommendations for when the patient should be evaluated in person.

If, however, after reading the patient e-communication significant additional history is needed, it is likely a situation in which an appointment (in-person, or telemedicine, depending on the concern) is indicated (Table 17.7).

Table 17.6 Examples of responding to patient messages in a manner that answers anticipated questions

Scenario	Patient message	Response by provider
Patient sends a follow-up message regarding blood pressure control after starting a new blood pressure medication	Dear Dr. ___, I've been on the amlodipine at 5 mg for 1 month now. I don't have any side effects. Attached are my blood pressure readings. What should we do next? Sincerely, [Patient Name]	Dear [Patient Name], I have sent in a new prescription for amlodipine at a higher dose, 10 mg daily. Please schedule an appointment in 4–6 weeks so that we can follow up on your blood pressure management. Sincerely, [Provider Name]
Patient sends an EHR message regarding a lingering cough after an upper respiratory infection. In their message, they report they've been afebrile and otherwise feel well	Dear Dr. ___, I've been coughing for 2 weeks, even though my cold has passed. I don't have fevers and I guess I feel OK overall, but should I be worried about the cough? Sincerely, [Patient Name]	Dear [Patient Name], I'm glad to hear you aren't having fevers and are overall feeling well. A cough after a bad cold may linger for several weeks. If your cough is still bothering you after 4–6 weeks, please schedule a clinic appointment. If you develop a fever, difficulty in breathing, or other concerning symptoms, please contact our clinic staff for a more urgent assessment. Sincerely, [Provider Name]

Table 17.7 Examples of responding to patient concerns that are not ideally addressed via e-communication

Scenario	Patient-initiated e-communication	Provider (or care team) response
A patient is noted to have high blood pressure at another health-care setting (e.g., dentist's office) and sends an EHR message to the provider	Dear Dr. __: I was seen at my dentist's office last week and they said my blood pressure was too high. What should I do? Sincerely, [patient name]	Dear [patient name], Thank you for letting me know. I need to evaluate your blood pressure in an in-person appointment. If you have a home blood pressure machine, please start checking your home readings and bring a record of them to the visit. My staff will contact you to schedule an appt. Sincerely, [Provider Name]
A patient has new onset knee pain and sends an EHR message to the provider	Dear Dr. __: My right knee has started acting up. It is a bit swollen and sometimes hard to go upstairs. Should I get an X-ray? [Patient Name]	Dear [patient name], Thank you for letting me know. You may need an X-ray, but I should evaluate you in-person to do a thorough evaluation. Would you please contact my office to arrange an appointment? Sincerely, [Provider Name]

17.4.4 Greeting

It is generally recommended to have a greeting when writing to a patient via EHR messaging. Using no greeting is an option but may give the impression of being less polite. As with any written communication (such as letters, emails), there are three components to an opening line address:

- **Salutation** (e.g., Dear, Hello, Hi): In general, professional salutations should be used. "Dear" is a generally accepted greeting. Patients may write more informally ("Hi Doctor" or "Hey Dr. ___") and while it may be tempting to match their level of written language, it is better to err on the side of using professional language.
- **Personal titles** (e.g., Mr., Mrs., Ms., Dr.): Personal titles may be used if a patient initiates a message and signs their name using a personal title. They may also be used if they are known from personal knowledge of the patient, or if a health-care system's EHR data is accurate. However, as with pronouns, there are varied methods to obtain this data, and if the data is inaccurate, it can lead to non-gender-affirming care (see Chap. 4). If there is any uncertainty as to personal title, its use should be avoided altogether.
- **Name**: If a personal title is used, then typically the patient's last name would follow. If no personal title is used, then the patient's name as the patient prefers to be addressed should be used. The patient's preferred name may be known to the provider already; or it may be inferred if a patient initiates the message and signs with their first name only (if a patient signs with both their first and last name, one cannot be certain how they prefer to be addressed); or the health-care system may have obtained this information and recorded it in the EHR. If there is any uncertainty about a patient's preferred name, then opening with *Dear [First Name] [Last Name]* is a reasonable alternative.
  If in doubt about a patient's preferred name and personal title, it may also be an opportunity to ask the patient in an open manner. While gender is considered an innate characteristic and the term "preferred" should be avoided when referring to gender, names may still be considered as preferences.

17.4.5 Signature

E-communication does not always identify who on the care team is responding to the message. It is recommended that you include a signature including your professional title on any E-communication (e.g., *Sincerely, [First Name] [Last Name], MD* or *Thank you, Dr. [First Name] [Last Name]*).

17.4.6   Language and Tone

Language and tone can easily be misinterpreted in written communication. Keeping the response professional, brief, and using straightforward language may help avoid miscommunication. The increased use of electronic communication has changed language itself, including style of writing and punctuation. It is likely that interpretations of tone will continue to evolve and vary between people (For example, the period is sometimes interpreted as conveying a serious or upset tone in mobile phone text communications; the use of quotes has changed as well—see Chaps. 3 and 7). Informal expressions may be used, but the writer should take caution as they can be misinterpreted—for example, rather than writing *I think we should...* a better practice would be to make clear what the clinical impressions are: *I recommend....*

The patient-centered language best practices discussed in the previous chapters apply to e-communications as well.

In situations where a provider does not know the patient—for example, covering for a colleague who is not in the office—it is best to use a neutral greeting without assumptions of gender or personal title (see above), as well as introduce one's role: *I am a colleague of Dr. ____, helping care for their patients while they are temporarily out of the office.*

17.5   Difficult E-Communication Issues

17.5.1   Declining a Patient's Request

There will be times when a patient makes a request that you do not feel comfortable fulfilling. Maintaining a therapeutic relationship with the patient while acknowledging and declining their request can require thoughtful language, including the rationale for declining the patient's request, and the provider's suggested alternative approach, if applicable (Table 17.8). A common issue is not being able to adequately address a request via e-communication and recommending an appointment to evaluate.

As with verbal communications, not all patients will respond to all types of written communication styles. If the message exchange appears to be going poorly, it is generally better to switch to speaking directly with the patient.

17.5.2   Responding to E-Communications That Are Excessive in Number or Length

There will be times when a patient sends messages very frequently or messages that are very long, with many questions or symptoms embedded in them. In these situations, reviewing expectations of e-communication use can be helpful. This

Table 17.8 Declining a patient request

Scenario	Suggested language
Patient requests a prescription for antibiotics, concerned they have bacterial sinusitis	Dear ___, I'm sorry to hear that you are having sinus symptoms. In order to determine the best treatment for you, I recommend that you be evaluated in a clinic visit. Please call or use the patient portal to schedule an appointment. Thank you, Dr. _____
Patient requests a referral for a condition that you have not evaluated previously in clinic	Dear ___, I'm sorry to hear that you are having knee pain. Prior to placing a referral, I need to evaluate you in the clinic. We can discuss treatment options once I have a better understanding of your condition. Please call or use the patient portal to schedule an appointment. Thank you, Dr. _____

Table 17.9 Addressing long or frequent messages

Scenario	Suggested language
Very long message	Dear ____, After reading your message, I am concerned at the symptoms that you are experiencing. I will be unable to address them adequately through a message. Please schedule a clinic visit. Thank you, Dr. ____
Frequent messages	Dear ____, Over the past couple weeks, I have received several messages from you. Thank you for letting me know about your concerns. In order to best address them and to make sure that I am answering your questions clearly, please schedule a clinic visit. Thank you, Dr. _____

discussion is likely best held in person rather than through e-messaging to ensure understanding.

In situations where the behavior persists despite previous conversations, then setting clear limits and expectations should be considered. For example, you can advise the patient that you will not be able to respond to their messages more than once a week, or that you will read their message but only respond with brief messages indicating that you would like them to come into the clinic for an evaluation (Table 17.9). If there are concerns that a patient is not appropriately using e-communications—for example, using inappropriate language, or repeatedly sending messages about urgent symptoms that should be triaged by phone—then the provider should involve their local health-care system's leadership and follow their local policies and procedures.

17.5.3 Responding to a Patient's Concern About Their Care

E-communication is now another mechanism through which a patient may raise questions about their care, in addition to letters, phone calls, in-person discussions, and, where available, engagement with centralized offices such as Patient Relations (these resources vary by health-care system). If a patient raises concerns about the care they are receiving, it is best to avoid further discussion via e-communication.

Resources will vary based on the provider's clinic/institution. In a setting where there is a formal patient relations liaison, providing a patient with that resource can be helpful; in other situations, referring to a clinic manager to talk with the patient may be an option. If it is a concern about care that you delivered, it would also be appropriate to ask the patient to schedule a visit to discuss in person. If medicolegal issues are raised, then involving one's local legal and administrative resources for guidance is appropriate before responding. Examples are shown in Table 17.10.

17.5.4 Addressing Messages from People Other Than the Patient

There are many situations in which it is not unexpected that communication through a patient's EHR portal is written by a family member, such as the spouse or adult child of a patient with dementia or who has difficulty using technology. Some EHRs allow for that person to be formally named a patient's proxy, while others may not have that capability. It is more challenging to know what to do when communication from someone other than the patient is unexpected. How to best address this situation depends on the request. A request to schedule an appointment or refill a

Table 17.10 Responding to patient concerns about service or quality or care

Scenario	Suggested language
Patient concern about clinic policy: *The time frame for the response from your clinic is not acceptable. I needed to discuss these issues with someone yesterday and didn't get any information until today!*	*Dear _____,* *I'm sorry that you did not get a response as quickly as you wanted. If you would like to talk to our clinic manager about you concern, please call them at XXX-XXX-XXXX; we can also discuss this at your next clinic visit.* *Sincerely,* *Dr. ____*
Patient concern about care delivery: *When I was getting my chest x-ray after our visit, the people working there were rude.*	*Dear ____,* *I'm sorry to hear about this. There is a patient relations office at the medical center that you can report this to if you wish, their number is XXX-XXX-XXXX.* *Sincerely,* *Dr. ____*

Table 17.11 Responding to e-communications from an unexpected source

Scenario	Suggested response
Adult child sends message through their mother's chart with concern that their mother is depressed and needs to restart her antidepressant medication.	Dear ____, Thanks for making me aware of your concerns. Please encourage your mother to make a clinic appointment so that we can discuss this in person. Sincerely, Dr. ____

noncontrolled medication is likely reasonable, whereas a request to adjust a medication dose based on symptoms or information on new symptoms would need confirmation with the patient (Table 17.11). If there is any doubt, clinic staff should contact the patient to confirm that the other person writing has permission to speak (write) on the patient's behalf.

17.6   Telephone Call Documentation

Prior to the commonplace use of the EHR, telephone calls had varied documentation practices—brief notations in a paper chart, emails, or even no documentation at all for calls perceived as minor in nature. Since the advent of the EHR, telephone notes (sometimes called telephone encounters) have been a means for health-care professionals to efficiently communicate and document care conversations between clinicians and staff to address outpatient care needs outside of clinic appointments. In the case of sensitive topics such as intimate partner or domestic violence, nonvisible telephone encounters were at times intentionally used in case the abuser may have electronic access to the other parts of the medical record. Another scenario for the use of telephone encounter documentation was for clinicians discussing specific case scenarios with one another before deciding on a diagnosis or treatment plan. In the past, this documentation may have been in a telephone encounter before contacting a patient with a comprehensive plan. In some cases, reading these discussions prior to talking with their providers about the concern can be very sensitive and potentially devastating to a patient if the diagnosis is serious.

However, in the United States, the 21st Century Cures Act was passed in 2016, and implemented in 2021, and as of October 6, 2022, nearly all parts of the medical chart are released to the patient, including telephone and refill encounters [13]. Thus, the same patient-centered communication principles discussed elsewhere in this book should apply to telephone and refill encounters documented in the EHR.

For cases that include sensitive information, such as intimate partner violence or discussion of concerning diagnoses, other options for documentation in the chart could be considered, such as staff messages that are not part of the patient's chart. If using a telephone encounter, a provider should consider whether it should be made "not visible" to a patient. As with clinic notes, an exception exists to prevent information sharing if the person writing the note believes that a patient will harm another person or themselves if they or others were to read the note. Clinicians will need to be attentive and mindful about actively turning off note sharing with the patient to prevent harm. If this decision is made to not share the information with the patient, the EHR will often be set up to prompt documentation of the rationale for not sharing the note. Consequently, when sensitive topics are discussed or serious illness may be identified, an upfront discussion with patients regarding wishes around documentation and release of results that are patient-viewable is helpful.

17.7   Challenging Telephone Communication Documentation Issues

17.7.1   New Serious Diagnosis but Unable to Reach the Patient on Telephone

With a new or concerning lab or imaging finding, it is clearly best to speak with the patient in person or by phone, but it can be challenging to reach them by telephone. In this case, there are several possible options regarding next steps. Keep in mind that if the patient uses their patient portal regularly, they may have already seen the results that were automatically released and be anxiously awaiting the provider's input. For patients who use the patient portal, and the provider is unable to connect with them on the telephone, sending them a follow-up electronic communication is an option. This also allows one to give the patient a message with sensitive information in a safe, private manner rather than on an answering machine, and to avoid unnecessary anxiety caused by waiting (Table 17.12).

17.7.2   Active Patient Care Discussions

Often a phone call is initiated by a patient or another member of a patient's care team calling into clinic with a question. There is then back-and-forth communications between staff and providers, which may be documented in the phone note before formally getting back to the patient—but it is important to recall that patients are able to view these communications and that the language should remain clear and professional, making sure to avoid words that could be misinterpreted (Table 17.13).

If there are complex discussions that need to occur between members of a patient's care team, it may be best to have these discussions over the phone or with clinic staff prior to documenting a summary in the patient chart. Some EHRs allow for private communication between the health-care team in a "staff message" function, which is not visible to the patient and not saved to the patient chart.

Table 17.12 Potentially serious results and telephone communication

Scenario	Possible courses of action and suggested language
You want to talk to a patient about the results of their chest CT. They have a spiculated mass concerning for a primary lung cancer. You have called twice but reached an answering machine without an identifying name on its message. You left a message to call back	Option 1
	If a patient does not use a patient portal and you are primarily using the telephone note for documentation that you called the patient and what you want your clinic team to be aware of if the patient calls back
	Telephone documentation:
	I left a voice mail message asking the patient to call me back at clinic. I would like to review their CT scan results with them by phone. If the patient calls back, please page me or ask for good times for me to call the patient back.
	Option 2
	If you suspect the patient may read your telephone note before you have a chance to connect with them by phone to discuss. Consider documenting findings and plan for follow-up in patient-centered language in the telephone encounter
	Telephone documentation:
	I left a voice mail message asking the patient to call me back at clinic. I would like to review his CT scan results with him by phone. The CT scan is concerning and needs further evaluation, and I would like to discuss the next steps, which may include...
	Option 3
	If the patient uses their patient portal, you can often see if they have viewed the result. Particularly, in that case, it would be reasonable to leave them a voice message that you are available to talk by telephone but will also send them a message through the patient portal, in this message describe what the findings may mean and next steps
	Telephone documentation:
	I sent the patient an electronic message about their CT scan results. Advised them to make a follow-up appointment to discuss next steps.
	E-communication:
	Dear _____, *I just left a message on your phone. I would like to talk to you about the results of your CT scan (lung images). As you may have seen in the test report, there is a mass in your lungs that is concerning for cancer and needs further evaluation. We will need to do further tests and involve other doctors in your care to determine the best next steps. Please call into clinic so that we can discuss the results, our number is XXX-XXX-XXXX, or if you prefer, you can message me back here.* *I know this kind of news can be stressful. I am available to answer any questions and support you through the next steps.* *Sincerely,* *Dr ____*

Table 17.13 Telephone calls and active care discussions

Scenario	Suggested strategies and language
Patient calling into clinic, requests antibiotics for a sinus infection, declines offer to schedule an appointment and asks for a prescription without a visit. History of similar requests, last visit >6 months ago. You are frustrated as you've discussed with the patient that they need an appointment in these situations	Avoid expressing frustration in your comments, keep language objective
	Please advise the patient that they need a clinic visit to discuss, in order to assure that we treat them with the best therapy. Please also encourage conservative measures
Gastroenterology clinic calls to ask how you want to handle patient's anticoagulation and antiplatelet medications prior to colonoscopy. These medications have been handled by patient's cardiologist; GI team notes the cardiology clinic has not responded to their requests. Procedure is in 5 days	Avoid making disparaging comments about other providers; keep the focus on taking the best care of the patient
	Depending on clinic resources this is a situation where calling—either the provider or an RN if available—the cardiology group to figure out the best course of action prior to documenting in the chart should be considered
	RN, please call cardiology clinic to discuss

17.8 Conclusion

Electronic communication in healthcare is undergoing rapid growth, due in part to the 21st Century Cures Act, OpenNotes, and the COVID-19 pandemic. Patient and health-care provider use of patient portals and e-communication have accelerated and the volumes of messages remain high. Learning to use this technology to improve patient care is critically important. Patient-centered language and the skills used to communicate effectively need to be applied to e-communication as well as verbal communication with patients. Health-care systems are recognizing the time this new component of patient care takes and are developing processes to reimburse for it [14]. Medicine is in constant evolution, not only with new developments in diagnostics and therapeutics, but also in care delivery. Learning the skills of patient-centered e-communication is valuable and will require training for all health-care professionals who write notes, education for patients, and resource allocation by health-care systems.

References

1. Holmgren AJ, Downing NL, Tang M, Sharp C, Longhurst C, Huckman RS. Assessing the impact of the COVID-19 pandemic on clinician ambulatory electronic health record use. J Am Med Inform Assoc. 2022;29(3):453–60.
2. Sinsky CA, Shanafelt TD, Ripp JA. The electronic health record inbox: recommendations for relief. J Gen Intern Med. 2022;37(15):4002–3. https://doi.org/10.1007/s11606-022-07766-0.
3. Yang R, Zeng K, Jiang Y. Prevalence, factors, and association of electronic communication use with patient-perceived quality of care from the 2019 Health Information National Trends

Survey 5-cycle 3: exploratory study. J Med Internet Res. 2022;24(2):e27167. https://doi.org/10.2196/27167.

4. Lee WW, Sulmasy LS, American College of Physicians Ethics, Professionalism and Human Rights Committee. American College of Physicians Ethical guidance for electronic patient-physician communication: aligning expectations. J Gen Intern Med. 2020;35(9):2715–20. https://doi.org/10.1007/s11606-020-05884-1.

5. Clarke MA, Fruhling AL, Sitorius M, Windle TA, Bernard TL, Windle JR. Impact of age on patients' communication and technology preferences in the era of meaningful use: mixed methods study. J Med Internet Res. 2020;22(6):e13470. https://doi.org/10.2196/13470.

6. Mackert M, Mabry-Flynn A, Champlin S, Donovan EE, Pounders K. Health literacy and health information technology adoption: the potential for a new digital divide. J Med Internet Res. 2016;18(10):e264. https://doi.org/10.2196/jmir.6349.

7. Lyles CR, Nelson EC, Frampton S, Dykes PC, Cemballi AG, Sarkar U. Using electronic health record portals to improve patient engagement: research priorities and best practices. Ann Intern Med. 2020;172(11 Suppl):S123–9. https://doi.org/10.7326/M19-0876.

8. Carini E, Villani L, Pezzullo AM, Gentili A, Barbara A, Ricciardi W, Boccia S. The impact of digital patient portals on health outcomes, system efficiency, and patient attitudes: updated systematic literature review. J Med Internet Res. 2021;23(9):e26189. https://doi.org/10.2196/26189.

9. Han HR, Gleason KT, Sun CA, Miller HN, Kang SJ, Chow S, Anderson R, Nagy P, Bauer T. Using patient portals to improve patient outcomes: systematic review. JMIR Hum Factors. 2019;6(4):e15038. https://doi.org/10.2196/15038.

10. Yan Q, Jiang Z, Harbin Z, Tolbert PH, Davies MG. Exploring the relationship between electronic health records and provider burnout: a systematic review. J Am Med Inform Assoc. 2021;28(5):1009–21. https://doi.org/10.1093/jamia/ocab009.

11. Rittenberg E, Liebman JB, Rexrode KM. Primary care physician gender and electronic health record workload. J Gen Intern Med. 2022;37(13):3295–301. https://doi.org/10.1007/s11606-021-07298-z.

12. Alpert JM, Dyer KE, Lafata JE. Patient-centered communication in digital medical encounters. Patient Educ Couns. 2017;100(10):1852–8. https://doi.org/10.1016/j.pec.2017.04.019.

13. The Office of the National Coordinator for Health Information Technology. Cures Act final rule: information blocking exceptions. https://www.healthit.gov/sites/default/files/page2/2020-03/InformationBlockingExceptions.pdf. Accessed 26 Mar 2023.

14. Holmgren AJ, Byron ME, Grouse CK, Adler-Milstein J. Association between billing patient portal messages as e-visits and patient messaging volume. JAMA. 2023;329(4):339–42. https://doi.org/10.1001/jama.2022.24710.

Afterword

Christopher J. Wong and Sara L. Jackson

In this book, we have tried to do something that healthcare professionals rarely, if ever, have the luxury to do in the course of their day—reflect and think carefully about the words we choose when we write in the medical chart.

Opening notes to patients has led to our "bedside manner" needing a written counterpart. Our spoken words have always mattered, but so too does our writing. Without the benefit of tone of voice, eye contact, small talk, and physical gestures, the written word carries a greater burden to convey all that it is tasked to do.

While it may seem difficult at first to unlearn and relearn the writing we do countless times each day, the preceding chapters have shown that often simple changes in word choice and phrasing can elevate our written language from stigmatization to empowerment, from distrust to respect.

We may think of ourselves as merely note writers, but all who write about patients are also *authors*. We as authors of our patients' clinical journeys bear the responsibility to write with truth, fairness, and compassion.

As is so common in healthcare, what is good for patients is also good for healthcare professionals. As note transparency gives more agency to patients, so too should clinicians take back their notes. We can choose to be burned out by note writing, or we can decide to take the opportunity to return to what is important and write notes that restore patients as the central focus.

C. J. Wong · S. L. Jackson
Division of General Internal Medicine, Department of Medicine, University of Washington, Seattle, WA, USA

© The Editor(s) (if applicable) and The Author(s), under exclusive license to Springer Nature Switzerland AG 2023
C. J. Wong, S. L. Jackson (eds.), *The Patient-Centered Approach to Medical Note-Writing*, https://doi.org/10.1007/978-3-031-43633-8

Regulatory bodies can assist by reducing unnecessary documentation burdens. Our medical education culture can stop teaching writing traditions that lack value, are harmful, or both. Healthcare systems can facilitate patient engagement so that healthcare professionals stay up to date on changes in language.

Language will continue to evolve in ways that surprise us; curiosity and openness must guide us into the next stage of being co-authors of our patients' lives.

Index

© The Editor(s) (if applicable) and The Author(s), under exclusive license to
Springer Nature Switzerland AG 2023
C. J. Wong, S. L. Jackson (eds.), *The Patient-Centered Approach to Medical
Note-Writing*, https://doi.org/10.1007/978-3-031-43633-8

GPSR Compliance

The European Union's (EU) General Product Safety Regulation (GPSR) is a set of rules that requires consumer products to be safe and our obligations to ensure this.

If you have any concerns about our products, you can contact us on ProductSafety@springernature.com

In case Publisher is established outside the EU, the EU authorized representative is:

Springer Nature Customer Service Center GmbH
Europaplatz 3
69115 Heidelberg, Germany

Batch number: 10091867

Printed by Printforce, the Netherlands